ADVANCE PRAISE FOR *GIFTS FROM THE POOR*

"The great teacher Kahlil Gibran reminds us that love disappears when it is held too tightly, but comes back many times over when it is given away. I have seen Glenn Geelhoed live this truth as a superb teacher himself, and as a student and a healer as well. Glenn gives so generously of his talents and treasure on international medical missions. He moves among cultures and people as an equalizer, seeing differences not as obstacles but as opportunities. The joy of this book is the opportunity it gives us to learn from Glenn and with him."

—JAMIL SHAMI, PhD, president, Middle East Division, American Higher Education, Inc.

"Glenn Geelhoed epitomizes the ideal of life-long learning. I have heard the excitement in the voices of his students as they tell me about the experiences they have shared with him on medical missions: a curiosity about the world, awe at its wonders, and respect for its peoples and cultures; the positive force of energy and dedication; and a 'just do it' attitude about overcoming obstacles. Those who accompany Glenn come back with a profound understanding of how one individual's efforts can change the lives of many. Glenn shares that life-affirming message with all of us in his new book, *Gifts from the Poor*."

—DR. PATRICIA LATHAM, MD, associate professor of pathology and medicine, The George Washington University School of Medicine and Health Sciences

"In *Gifts from the Poor*, readers will meet the Glenn Geelhoed I've known since we were residents together in the 1960s: inquisitive, committed to excellence, a skillful surgeon, and an artful communicator. In the decades since, through the medical mission work we've both pursued, Glenn has taught much, learned even more, and brought back a wealth of remarkable stories and insights. What a joy it is to tag along on his travels and drink in his experiences through the pages of this book."

—DOUGLAS W. SODERDAHL, MD, FACS, founder and president, Global Medical Education, Inc.

"Glenn Geelhoed could have excelled as an academic surgeon in Washington, DC. Instead, he has made the 'bottom billion' of the planet his patients, and encouraged medical students to expand their horizons with him on his worldwide missions to care for the poor. Read this and be inspired."

—RICK HODES, MD, MACP; medical director, American Jewish Joint Distribution Committee; subject of the book *This is a Soul: the Mission of Rick Hodes* by Marilyn Berger

"In my work around the world on health care, from the White House to Haiti to Afghanistan, I've seen countless opportunities for the more fortunate people of the world to promote health for the less fortunate. No one is more committed to that mission than Glenn Geelhoed, who pours his time and talent into global medical service. With this book of colorful stories and powerful lessons, he calls the rest of us to find our own ways to serve."
—PAUL T. ANTONY, MD, MPH; executive director, Global Health Progress; Commander, U.S. Navy Medical Corps

"Two words describe this doctor-to-the-world: Inspired, and inspiring. Glenn Geelhoed is a role model for patients and peers alike. His energy and expertise are well recognized, day after day. So many, young and old, are his beneficiaries!"
—JOHN P. HOWE III, MD, president and CEO, Project HOPE

"When the American College of Surgeons presented Dr. Glenn Geelhoed with its Surgical Volunteerism Award for international outreach, we honored one man's unflagging commitment to providing surgical care and education throughout the world. As a physician and a teacher, Glenn has influenced generations of medical students and colleagues. With *Gifts from the Poor*, he continues and expands this great cause of his life: to raise awareness of the needs of a hurting world and to inspire others to join him in healing it. Glenn's story is an invitation to engaged global citizenship, and a testament to the power of humanitarianism in action."
—LaMAR S. McGINNIS JR., MD, FACS; president, American College of Surgeons; past president, American Cancer Society

"When I came to the United States as a 'Lost Boy' fleeing war-torn Sudan, I learned how generous Americans can be to people in great need. When I returned to Sudan to build a clinic in my home village, many generous, supportive people stood with me—among them, Dr. Geelhoed. He gave tirelessly of his talent and knowledge, treating our sick and training our Sudanese staff to provide care. As I have been privileged to know him in life, fortunate readers now may know him through this wise, inspiring book."
—JOHN BUL DAU, author of the memoir and subject of the documentary *God Grew Tired of Us*, a Grand Jury Prize Winner at the 2006 Sundance Film Festival

"Glenn Geelhoed thinks of himself as a learner, not a teacher, his textbook being the thousands of impoverished peoples in the darkest corners of the world whom he restlessly visits to deliver surgical care. This modern-day Pied Piper brings along a retinue of other learners who sign up to be volunteer caregivers but wind up awakening to an unimagined side of life. He impacts not only the patients he treats but also the multitudes who will be treated by his followers. True to the literal meaning of 'doctor' (teacher) despite his demurral, his influence will extend down through generations to come, through the legacy of his work and this book."

—ANDREW L. WARSHAW, MD, FACS, professor of surgery, Harvard Medical School; surgeon-in-chief, Massachusetts General Hospital; founder, Operation Giving Back, American College of Surgeons

"In the neediest corners of the world, countless patients and practitioners have benefited from Glenn Geelhoed's wonderful gifts as a surgeon and a teacher. Now those people will benefit from Glenn's equal gifts as a chronicler, as he shares their life stories along with his own in *Gifts from the Poor*. Most of us never will do or see even a fraction of what Glenn has done and seen through scores of medical missions. But from the stories he shares in this compelling book, we can begin to learn what he has learned about the indomitability of the human spirit, and the power of each individual to shape a better world."

—LaSalle D. Leffall Jr., MD, FACS; dean emeritus of the Howard University School of Medicine; author of *No Boundaries: A Cancer Surgeon's Odyssey*

Gifts

from the
Poor

What the World's Patients Taught One Doctor About Healing

DR. GLENN W. GEELHOED
with PATRICIA EDMONDS

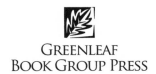

GREENLEAF
BOOK GROUP PRESS

Published by Greenleaf Book Group Press
Austin, Texas
www.gbgpress.com

Distributed by Greenleaf Book Group LLC

For ordering information or special discounts for bulk purchases, please contact Greenleaf Book Group LLC at PO Box 91869, Austin, TX 78709, 512.891.6100.

Design and composition by Greenleaf Book Group LLC
Cover design by Greenleaf Book Group LLC
Photography by Dr. Glenn W. Geelhoed except where noted

Publisher's Cataloging-In-Publication Data
(Prepared by The Donohue Group, Inc.)
Geelhoed, Glenn W., 1942–
  Gifts from the poor : what the world's patients taught one doctor about healing / Glenn W. Geelhoed and Patricia Edmonds.—1st ed.
   p. : ill. ; cm.
  ISBN: 978-1-60832-094-3
  1. Geelhoed, Glenn W., 1942– 2. Missions, Medical. 3. Missionaries, Medical—Biography. I. Edmonds, Patricia. II. Title.
R722.32.G44 G44 2011
610.69/092 B   2010940334

Part of the Tree Neutral® program, which offsets the number of trees consumed in the production and printing of this book by taking proactive steps, such as planting trees in direct proportion to the number of trees used: www.treeneutral.com

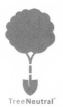
TreeNeutral®

Printed in the United States of America on acid-free paper

10 11 12 13 14 15   10 9 8 7 6 5 4 3 2 1

First Edition

Contents

PREFACE   ix

INTRODUCTION   1

FOREWORD   3

CHAPTER ONE: This Little Light of Mine   7

CHAPTER TWO: One Small Room in a Giant Mansion   13

CHAPTER THREE: Imagination and Organization   25

CHAPTER FOUR: Beyond "Medical Center Civilization"   35

CHAPTER FIVE: "Just Keep Operating and Learning"   45

CHAPTER SIX: Around Barriers and Over Bridges   57

CHAPTER SEVEN: Riding More than One Horse   71

CHAPTER EIGHT: The Year of Fulbrightness   81

CHAPTER NINE: The Gift of Deprivation   97

CHAPTER TEN: From Suffering, the Gift of Strength   109

CHAPTER ELEVEN: Cultures, Consonants and Vowels   123

CHAPTER TWELVE: Bricking Up the Leper Door   139

CHAPTER THIRTEEN: The Hunter-Gatherer and The Runner   155

CHAPTER FOURTEEN: Humility in Health Care   179

CHAPTER FIFTEEN: Hither by Thy Help   191

CHAPTER SIXTEEN: Transformation   207

CHAPTER SEVENTEEN: Giving Back   227

CHAPTER EIGHTEEN: Derwood   249

ACKNOWLEDGMENTS   259

Preface

The Medical Mission Hall of Fame Foundation, based at the University of Toledo, is proud to partner with Dr. Glenn Geelhoed in the creation of this book.

The Medical Mission Hall of Fame (www.medicalmissionhalloffame-foundation.org) was founded in 2002 to honor individuals and organizations that significantly advance the health and well-being of people around the world through medical mission activities. Individual Hall of Fame awards are presented to physicians, nurses and other medical providers to honor their humanitarian service. Institutional Hall of Fame awards are presented to groups, associations and corporations that lend financial or other support to medical mission endeavors.

By providing medical care and training, public-health education, social-welfare services, and medical equipment, supplies and technology, Hall of Fame honorees have brought health and hope to people on every continent. The Foundation, a 501 c (3) organization, assists these honorees and other mission endeavors with travel stipends, equipment and supply donations, and organizational and logistical support. The Foundation's work is funded through private contributions, grants, endowments and legacies of individuals and organizations.

Glenn Geelhoed, a Medical Mission Hall of Fame Award recipient in 2005, stands as a shining of example of what this organization seeks to exalt:

selfless humanitarian efforts that heal and inspire. Glenn continues his long tradition of support and service to the Hall of Fame by making it the recipient of the proceeds from sales of this book, *Gifts from the Poor*. On behalf of the Medical Mission Hall of Fame Foundation and the University of Toledo, we thank him for his generosity. And we pledge our continued support of Glenn's work, which can be followed at his web site, www.MissionToHeal.org.

—LAWRENCE V. CONWAY, PhD
   President, Medical Mission Hall of Fame Foundation

—JEFFREY P. GOLD, MD
   Dean, College of Medicine Provost, The University of Toledo

—LLOYD A. JACOBS, MD
   President, The University of Toledo

INTRODUCTION

FROM 1958 TO 1973, I GREW UP IN A MISSIONARY FAMILY ON THE SLOPES
of Mt. Kilimanjaro in Tanzania. My mother Jerene established the International School there; and my father Dempsey was the founder of Kilimanjaro Christian Medical Center (KCMC). In everything they did, my parents strove to empower the local people with two of the greatest forces for good that they knew: learning and healing.

I was nine when Dad gave me a book to read: *Reverence for Life*, by a medical missionary named Albert Schweitzer. Dr. Schweitzer's message—that we must treat all living beings as sacred—had a profound influence on my life. Over the years, a steady stream of medical missionaries visited KCMC. They came to serve patients and share their medical knowledge. They went away changed, their hearts and eyes opened to the needs of a hurting world. One of those visitors was Glenn Geelhoed.

In the four decades since we met, Glenn has forged paths of healing, leading medical missions to treat patients and train practitioners throughout the developing world. I have done what I can to foster learning, helping the people of Pakistan and Afghanistan build schools to educate their children, boys and especially girls. Glenn and I both work in partnership with real heroes: brave and inspiring people who strive—with meager resources and at great personal cost—to bring education and health care to their neighbors. Our faces, faiths and garbs may be different but our mission is the same: To promote peace and healing.

Glenn's book, *Gifts from the Poor*, bears a message for the world about the power of compassion and humility. I commend the incredible work Glenn does. May God bless him a hundred times over.

—GREG MORTENSON,
   coauthor of the international bestseller *Three Cups of Tea*

FOREWORD

EVER SINCE I WAS KID I HAVE WANTED TO STUDY THE DISEASES THAT afflict the world's poorest people, the so-called "bottom billion." In 2000 I came to the George Washington University (GWU) to focus on developing drugs and vaccines for these neglected tropical diseases (NTDs), parasitic and bacterial infections that include hookworm, schistosomiasis and river blindness. Tourists traveling abroad don't see these diseases because they're concentrated in the poorest, rural areas of countries throughout Africa, Asia and Latin America. Global policy makers take less notice because these diseases aren't always killers—but since they debilitate, deform and blind, they destroy people's ability to work and learn, which also destroys their ability to better themselves and their families.

I often describe these as forgotten diseases among forgotten people. But shortly after I arrived at GWU, I met a man who knows these diseases well, and has chosen these forgotten people as his patients.

Glenn Geelhoed's office is down the hall from mine, and upon my arrival at GWU, he came by to introduce himself. I was fascinated by him because I hadn't heard of his work before then. The work he was doing sounded tremendous. It was at a different end of the spectrum from what I'm doing at GWU and with the Sabin Vaccine Institute—we're on the research-and-development end of things, making new tools for controlling neglected diseases and shaping policy to ensure that the bottom billion have access to essential medicines for neglected diseases, while he's on the front lines, going all over the world.

Many things about Glenn impress me. There's his fearlessness—his ability to go into any area of the world, no matter how difficult. All of the places he has visited are resource-poor settings, yet he doesn't think twice about going, even into areas where there are conflicts. There's his adaptability—although he tries to go on these missions with the equipment and supplies that will be needed, he never knows quite what he'll be faced with, but he's still prepared to operate and do what needs to be done. There's his energy—if he's not operating or training for a marathon, then he's on a plane to do one or both. He'll go from Mindanao to Central Asia to sub-Saharan Africa, not thinking twice; he'll be home for a few days and be ready to go out again. How he does that, I don't know.

What really stands out about Glenn, though, is his love of teaching. He never goes on these missions alone; he always has a flock of students, residents and colleagues eager to learn. He's a great teacher, and a great role model. He's not doing this for money or glory. He does this, at some personal sacrifice, to make a difference in the world. At a time when the global health community talks a lot about how to address the lack of medical personnel in the developing world, Glenn is there, training his students who often return to serve—but more importantly, training locals who'll be there after he's gone.

Other people who lead medical missions have created organizations, traveled repeatedly to a single place and built an operation there. Glenn has chosen instead to go wherever the need is greatest, to do God's work on a person-by-person basis. No slave to structure, he's a bit of a maverick—and as a result, institutions, including our university, don't always know what to do with him. But the students somehow find out about him. We all find out about him. And when we do, we stand amazed at the difference he has made for the world's poorest patients, and are inspired to go do likewise.

—PROFESSOR PETER HOTEZ, MD, PHD

Dr. Peter Hotez is Distinguished Research Professor, the Walter G. Ross Professor and the chair of the Department of Microbiology, Immunology and Tropical Medicine at The

George Washington University, Washington, D.C. He is also president of the Sabin Vaccine Institute, a nonprofit medical research and advocacy organization. Through the Institute, Dr. Hotez founded the Human Hookworm Vaccine Initiative, a partnership supported by the Bill and Melinda Gates Foundation, to develop a vaccine for human hookworm disease. He also cofounded the Global Network for Neglected Tropical Diseases, sponsor of the Just 50 Cents campaign to control NTDs in developing countries.

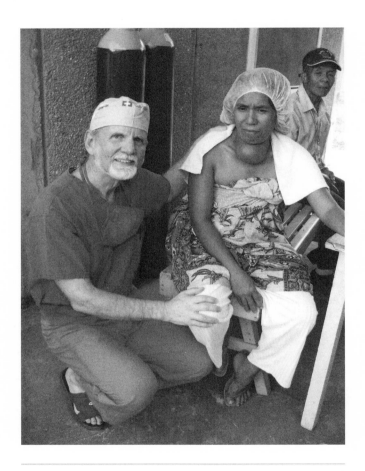

In South Cotabato on the island of Mindanao in the Philippines, Glenn poses with a thyroidectomy patient, one of fifteen whose goiters would be removed on the first surgical day of Glenn's January 2009 medical mission there.

CHAPTER ONE

This Little Light of Mine

DR. GLENN GEELHOED BENT OVER THE SLEEPING PATIENT, STITCHING closed a long incision. In the operating room of the Far North Luzon General Hospital, the surgeon worked at one of three tightly packed operating tables, the better to banter with colleagues. They were nurses, technicians and medical students, of all ages and backgrounds. Some were recruited and trained by Glenn for this medical mission to remote Apayo, one of the Philippines' poorest provinces.

Several volunteers were on their first such trip. Glenn was on his second of the month, having flown directly from the Sudan. Over four decades he had logged scores of missions, all driven by his medical mantra: "I will treat anyone anywhere any time, so long as they cannot pay."

Once word-of-mouth overcame disbelief—Yes, *duktors* doing operations for free!—the locals formed long lines outside the hospital, waiting for hours, even days, to be seen. By sundown on the third day, Glenn and the nine-person team already had done thirty-seven major operations and three times as many minor ones.

As Glenn completed hernia repairs, colleagues readied his next case, a patient sedated for gallbladder removal. On the second table, a patient

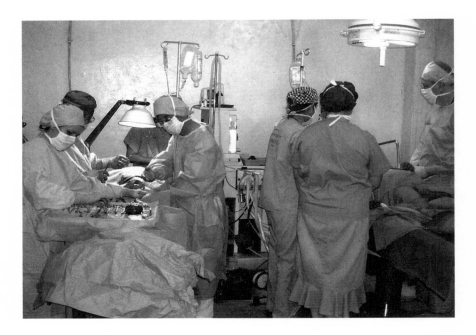

Glenn photographed the side-by-side tables where he and medical mission colleagues work in the operating room of the Far North Luzon General Hospital in the Philippines.

awaited a thyroidectomy to remove a grapefruit-sized goiter from her neck. And at the third table, a retired Akron, Ohio, surgeon named Alfredo Casino prepared to repair the cleft lip that had left an eighteen-year-old boy disfigured since birth.

For an instant, the operating room lights flared brighter. Then they went out. Accustomed to such glitches, Glenn fished in the darkness for his mountain climber's headlamp and clicked it on. In the weak light, the team debated what to do.

The woozy gallbladder patient could be walked into the recovery room and, since all beds were full, consigned to a chair. The eighteen-year-old already was anesthetized, but the cleft lip operation would be tricky without electric-powered cautery and suction instruments. Better to wait, at least for a while, and see if the power returned.

In the dim light from the headlamp, only those closest to him saw a smile cross Glenn's face. Then he began to sing, in a cheery if imperfect baritone: "This little light of mine, I'm going to let it shine." He had learned the song in Sunday school, during an all-American boyhood in Grand Rapids, Michigan. He sang it now, decades later, as a globetrotting physician-anthropologist bent on caring for and learning from the poorest people in the world.

"Let it shine, let it shine, let it shine." As Glenn's voice floated out from the operating room, others in the darkened wards joined in: surgeons, orderlies, patients tethered to IVs, waiting their turn. After a few choruses that he praised for their "rather impressive harmonies," Glenn struck up new tunes: the centuries-old Christian doxology and then "Amazing Grace." As they sang, people moved haltingly through the hospital, finding what lights they could: flashlights, headlamps, candles.

From the recovery room, a nurse called out: A patient whose thyroid gland had been removed earlier in the day was coughing and gasping for air. Bumping through the dark, the team returned the woman to the operating room. Power or no power, surgeons would have to reopen the eight-inch-long incision at the collar line of her neck.

With his headlamp trained on the patient, Glenn and colleagues moved swiftly. They opened the sutures, removing pooled blood that caused the distress, and were reclosing the incision just as the lights came back on. The patient stabilized and later made a full recovery. The team performed another twenty-nine operations before stopping at Glenn's idea of "an early closing time," about 11:00 p.m.

Midnight found the surgeon in a hospital ward turned makeshift dormitory, stretched out on the floor on a sleeping mat, not closing his eyes, but opening his laptop computer. Glenn's one constant in all his pursuits— practicing medicine or running marathons, hunting big game or collecting academic degrees—is to write relentlessly about these events almost as they occur.

Glenn cannot recall the last day he let pass unchronicled. Events, people and insights are meticulously documented, in text files on his high-mileage laptop or, when there's paper but not power, in dense, tiny handwriting. From the long day seeing patients in Apayo, his wrap-up included the following:

A complete power failure, not just in the OR, but in the entire district of Luna. People were calling out to ask if there was a generator, or to call the mayor, or for a number of absurd requests, as though they alone were inconvenienced by the blackout . . . I reminded them (after our harmonious songfest) that this is how I had operated for the last three weeks in the Sudan, without power or plumbing. We are now getting used to electricity and feel like we are out of business when we do not have it as a necessity rather than a privilege taken for granted—one of very many . . .

"What we did learn later is that the power outage came from two men who were electrocuted in the process of doing something to a transmission line. So we and our patients—even including the emergency reoperation in the dark—all did better than the two men who interrupted the electricity in the first place.

Alfredo Casino chuckles when recalling the late-night laptop typing, the operating-room sing-along, and the other memories he has from ten years of working with Glenn on medical missions. For Casino—a septuagenarian whose grandfatherly demeanor earned him the nickname "Poppy"—the missions are both payback and homecomings to his native Philippines.

Casino was once like those he now treats, a poor child plowing rice fields behind a water buffalo. "I know how it is to live in the barrios, how people just die because there is no doctor," he says. He made it through medical school and then on to the United States and a successful surgical practice. In retirement, eager to give back, he found a kindred spirit in Geelhoed: "He has such a missionary heart, not only to help poor people but to help medical students learn how it is in these Third World countries."

After a fourth flat-out day providing care at Far North Luzon hospital, Glenn moved on. His team spent the next week operating in the southern Philippine island of Mindanao, in an area many aid groups won't enter because anti-government Islamic rebels operate there.

Before 2009 ended, he would take mission trips to three more countries, plan several future promised trips, and add more names to the roster of hundreds of students and colleagues who have traveled and served with him.

When inviting people to join him, Glenn issues what can sound like a warning, or a promise—or, he might say, some of both. "This is an excursion beyond borders of all kinds and will have you superseding your own limits," he wrote to one recruit. "You will be kept busy in the most intensive learning experience of your life. You will return lighter (since I know some good running trails around where we will be). And you will return wiser, since you will see how most people of this planet cope with their struggles of everyday living!"

Everything Glenn does to foster medical missions—booking and bankrolling travel, recruiting clinicians, and gathering supplies—he does in the name of learning. Others join in because they want to serve, to heal, to teach, to train under Glenn, and he does not dissuade them. But he hopes that by a mission's end they see these endeavors more as he does. The teachers, he insists, are not the drop-in doctors. The teachers are the cultures themselves, the environments, the experiences, and, above all, the world's impoverished patients. "The rest of us," he says, "are just learners."

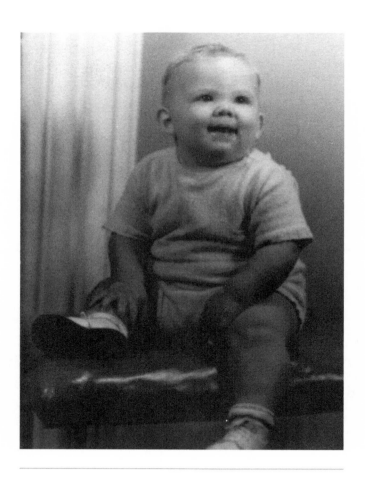

Glenn William Geelhoed's baby portrait, 1942.

CHAPTER TWO

One Small Room in a Giant Mansion

GLENN GEELHOED'S DERWOOD, MARYLAND, HOME IS JAMMED WITH souvenirs from his travels. In the living room, stacking Matrushka dolls from Russia share shelf space with fish scales from a mammoth Amazonian *pirarucu* and carved wooden god figures from Cambodia. A 3,000-year-old Egyptian painting on papyrus hangs near a trio of samurai swords in red silk sheaths. One glass case holds mementoes from all seven continents, including a painted Andean figure from Chile, a polished malachite box from the Congo, and an alabaster vase from Kashmir.

Alongside treasures from the places he has gone, Glenn keeps a prized artifact of where he came from. It is a battered, child-sized wooden desk from Southwest Christian Elementary School in Grand Rapids, Michigan. On the desk's pencil-scarred surface, a gangly, inquisitive boy once spread out library copies of *National Geographic* and drank in the exotic scenes. Today Glenn chuckles at the seeming distance between his "happy, unexceptional childhood" and his globe-spanning later life. But in many ways he still is rooted to that home place, through family, tradition and history.

It was in the final months of the nineteenth century that William Geelhoed was born. He joined three siblings and was followed by four more, two sisters and six brothers in all. Carefully preserved family photos capture Bill as a young man: a rakish figure in a straw boater, taking young ladies out for rowboat rides on the lake.

A smart and diligent student, Bill long dreamt of college but left school after eighth grade to help his parents pay the bills. Bill was twenty-four when he met Alice Stuk, a year younger than he. The middle child of nine, Alice was a fine-featured young woman with an unfailingly sunny outlook despite a dislocated hip that gave her a lifelong, painful limp.

After a quick and chaperoned courtship, Bill and Alice married. The young newlyweds took their place in the familiar circles of west Michigan life: big families filling Christian Reformed Church pews, mothers tending kids and gardens, fathers working for tool-and-die companies, auto parts suppliers or furniture manufacturers. Grand Rapids so regarded itself as "the Furniture City" that the call letters for a local radio station were WFUR, and the TV station was WOOD.

Bill and Alice bought a modest house on Hall Street, with a big yard and garden and a decal in the window reminding the ice man to leave blocks for the icebox. Daughter Martheen was born in 1932, and Shirley two and a half years later. For eight years, no more babies arrived as the little family scrimped its way through the Depression. In the bitter cold of January 1942, Alice went to Butterworth Hospital to bear her son, Glenn William. While the middle name was supplied by the baby's proud father, unconfirmed family lore credits Alice with selecting Glenn, the name of a long-ago beau.

The birth day of his son, January 19, was Bill Geelhoed's first day on the job at the Kindel Furniture Company, one of the seven guild companies that made Grand Rapids a center of U.S. furniture manufacturing. Though Bill always would call himself "just a shipping clerk," he oversaw everything that came into or went out of the bustling company, including, during World War II, parts for wooden glider planes that played a major role in the Normandy invasion on D-day.

The arrival of baby Milly in 1943 completed the family—almost two separate generations of siblings as Glenn remembers it, teenaged sisters driving while he and Milly still were walking to school. Still, everyone in the family shared household chores, everyone worked in the big garden, and everyone helped grow tomatoes, which neither Glenn nor his father would eat.

When Alice couldn't can any more tomatoes and they overran the kitchen, she'd send Glenn up and down the street with his red wagon loaded with the produce. "People would look at me and say, 'Oh no, here he comes again,'" Glenn recalls. "At one point I set up a stand and was going to sell a half-peck basket for a nickel. But I was competing with myself, since I just had wheeled through the neighborhood giving them away."

The sales scheme never suited Alice, anyway. She would gently chide her son, "God's good earth gave us this. What would we be doing selling it?" It was typical of the mother Glenn knew: always looking for a way to give, asking what she could do to help. She would scrimp as she spent the weekly grocery allowance and put whatever she had left in a Mason jar saying, "Someone else may need this."

Bill Geelhoed was a sterner sort. Glenn's sisters still tell of the Thanksgiving when Glenn proudly roasted a turkey to be carved with ceremony at the table, and how, because Bill objected to his son's doing the cooking, their father refused to eat what Glenn had prepared. Once Bill formed a belief about something or someone, for good or ill, that was that.

At first young Glenn thought he'd like to have that same sense of unbending certitude, that legacy from his very religious ancestors, for whom divine revelation had trumped most other insights. But over time, as some of his father's convictions came to look more like prejudices or blind spots, Glenn saw his own goal a little differently. He aimed to thoughtfully form convictions while trying to see all sides; to hold to truths steadfastly but not rigidly.

As an adult, Glenn framed the whole question as a joke on himself: "I have many strongly held convictions, the strongest of which being that I might possibly be wrong." Still, says sister Shirley, the family legacy is clear: "It was hard for Dad to admit when he was wrong, and Glenn gets some of that from Dad."

Like virtually all in their extended clan and most in their neighborhood, Glenn's family attended the Christian Reformed Church, where his sisters remember him as "a model pew-sitter," well-behaved and quiet.

A denomination founded on scriptural truth as interpreted by Protestant reformer John Calvin, the CRC told members it was their duty to help transform the world. But it also warned members that much outside the church was "worldly" and to be approached cautiously if at all.

Glenn embraced the first teaching but not the second. To him, the unknown was inviting, not alarming. "As a kid, I was never out of Kent County," he recalls. "But when I went to the library and pulled out those *National Geographics*, pulled out that other world, I would wonder: Do all those people living in those places not know they're stuck in one small room in this giant mansion? What if we could get out and see all the other rooms?" Sister Milly recalls that when people asked Glenn what he wanted to be when he grew up, "he always said, 'a medical missionary.'" While he dreamed of venturing farther, Glenn intrepidly explored his corner of Kent County. With only girl siblings and not many boy playmates nearby, he spent a lot of time alone. He wandered for hours in the woods near his house and family friends' cottages, stalking as if on safari.

In winter in the woods, he played in snowfalls with drifts up to his chin. In fall, he kicked through blazing red leaves shed by towering maple and sassafras trees. In spring and summer, he liked to cut saplings and whittle sticks to make bows and arrows, and then creep up on rabbits or birds. "Many times I would draw back with the little homemade arrows, but I didn't often release because I didn't really want to kill them," he later recalled.

More often, he used the sticks as fishing poles. On his own in Grand Rapids, he'd bike five miles to little Fisk Lake, net a few minnows for bait, and then fish for crappie and bass. He once caught more fish than could be suspended from the bicycle frame, so he pedaled home with the bike wobbling under one load. Then he pedaled back for the second batch. When his dad could get away, they'd drive an hour to pull perch out of Lake Michigan, which to Glenn looked as big as an ocean.

"If I were invited on a fishing trip," he says, "it was assumed that I was the baiter of hooks, the taker-off of fish, and the fish cleaner. So I became an anatomist at a very early age." Never one to waste, he shared what he caught with the neighbors.

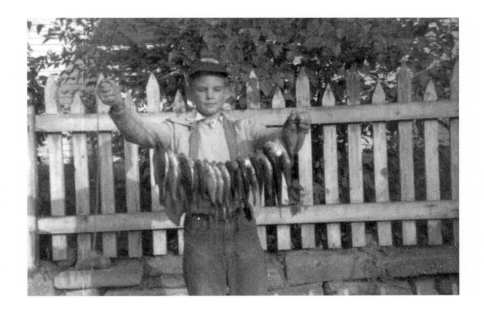

Glenn at age 13 with a stringer of fish he caught in Fisk Lake near his family's Grand Rapids, Michigan, home.

Glenn was fourteen before he ventured beyond Michigan, on a driving vacation with family. In 1956, during the one week of the year that Bill Geelhoed was granted for vacation, Glenn, Milly and parents piled into the Packard to visit newlywed Martheen and her husband, Donald Griffioen, a seminary student on summer assignment to a small church in rural Iowa.

Glenn remembers the exhilaration of crossing the Mississippi River, feeling like an explorer with a new land opening up before him. The sights were not exotic: a town square bounded by dirt roads and livestock yards, a Fourth of July fireworks show watched from blankets on the town park lawn. But they were new sights, new places to Glenn, and that alone made them memorable. "It made me feel like I had really stepped out into the world," he says.

In his own way, Bill Geelhoed was as eager to learn as his son was. Bill was among the first folks in west Michigan to have a Model A Ford. He was also among the first in town to have a television (though he insisted that the doors covering the tube remain closed on Sundays, the Lord's Day). The job at Kindel enabled Bill to support the family, but it left neither time nor money for one thing he longed to acquire: a college education.

When Stewart Geelhoed was finishing high school and looking for a path out of the poverty bred by the Depression, he asked his uncle Bill for advice on what course his life should take. Someone had given Bill a copy of *Prism*, the yearbook of the CRC-affiliated Calvin College. In a moment that would become cherished family legend, Bill gave the book to Stewart and urged, "Whatever you do, graduate from college—this college."

Stewart did just that, with his uncle's encouragement and the few dollars Bill could spare. He became the first in the Geelhoed family to earn his college degree and went on to success in business, first as a paper-company executive in Michigan and later at Nabisco, in New York City. A quarter century later, the second Geelhoed to graduate college was Martheen, who went on to get a master's in church education and then became one of the first two women to graduate from the Calvin Theological Seminary.

While his older sisters were teaching school, Glenn was in high school, hustling to keep his grades up while working after-school jobs. He stocked grocery shelves and delivered phoned-in orders. At a construction site, he lugged eighty-pound cement bags for sixty cents an hour, watching the clock and imagining one penny dropping into his paycheck every time the second hand passed twelve. One especially tiring shift, he asked himself the question out loud: "Are you going to spend the rest of your life watching pennies drop?" He resolved that in adulthood, insofar as he could help it, he never would do any job just for the money.

In 1960, when he graduated from Grand Rapids Christian High School with honors, his gifts and career interests led in two directions. Which should he choose: literature and philosophy, "the life of the mind," or science and medicine, a life of discovery and healing? Or maybe, somehow, both?

Glenn never seriously considered enrolling anywhere but Calvin College. By the time he started classes, in 1960, sisters Martheen and Shirley both were pursuing teaching careers, after earning master's degrees in education. As his sisters had before him, he raised the $3,600 for his annual

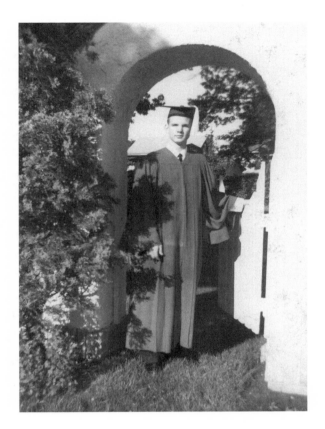

Glenn gowned for his 1960 graduation from Grand Rapids Christian High School.

tuition—a significant sum in those days, probably equal to half his father's annual take-home pay.

Like many Calvin students from Grand Rapids families, Glenn lived at home instead of on campus, to economize. When other freshmen were decorating their dorm-room walls with posters of the Beatles, he just moved some camping gear out of his childhood bedroom to make shelf space for his college books. At Calvin, Glenn shared a locker with Don Gabrielson, another premed student with whom he struck up a friendship.

The campus was one large city block, with a commons in the center; a student standing on one edge could see all the way to the others. If the surroundings were modest, the ambitions were not: Calvin was determined to foster intellectual rigor and outstanding scholarship as well as a Christian environment.

For its academics, Calvin earned praise as "the Notre Dame of the evangelical Protestant world." For atmospherics, it drew a more tongue-in-cheek appraisal: Sydney Youngsma, Calvin's first fulltime publicist, once called the college "a hotbed of decency, complacency and gentlemanliness." Under the leadership of president William Spoelhof, a revered educator and World War II hero, Calvin's quiet tradition of piety stood in contrast to the fundamentalism and spectacle at other evangelical institutions, the Billy Graham crusades and Oral Roberts healings.

Glenn's wry synopsis of his college career: "Instead of drinking and chasing women, I was a good little worker bee." In his one splurge from the college store, a red-leather-covered binder stamped with the school emblem, he tracked every assignment, class and task. The Calvin administration considered eighteen course hours per semester a fulltime academic load; Glenn often took twenty-four course hours, sometimes more. He took careful class notes but seldom consulted them before tests, finding—as he would throughout his life—that the act of writing something down lodged it firmly in his memory. He almost never missed a class, reasoning that each one represented a chunk of his hard-earned dollars.

After classes, he would walk the few miles into East Grand Rapids to Blodgett Memorial Hospital, where he worked several shifts a week. He started as an orderly, transporting patients back and forth for X-rays, and then worked his way into the emergency room. Blodgett's physicians and nurses appreciated the college kid's quick grasp of what he observed, his enthusiasm and eagerness to pitch in. "Oh, can I do that?" he was forever asking. Before long he was scrubbing in to observe operations and even doing simple sutures.

Between working, studying and living at home, Glenn had little time to cultivate campus friendships. Some days his only socializing was running into Don at their locker, where the two premed students would compare notes about papers and tests. Glenn remembers hearing through the grapevine that Don had a girlfriend. He planned to ask him about it when they next met. But while Don was home for the summer in Cadillac, Michigan, doctors discovered he had lymphoma and told him that the cancer was inoperable.

Within a few years, revolutions in drug therapy would make lymphoma one of the most treatable, survivable cancers, especially with young patients. But Don did not have years. Glenn never again saw Don; he died at age 20, at the start of what would have been his senior year. The abruptness of Don's death haunted Glenn. *Gone before I could ask about that girl*, he remembers thinking. *Gone before I really got to know him.*

Powering through his premed courses and learning medicine on the job at Blodgett, Glenn still longed to explore the humanities so he took those courses as well. "I liked the idea of being a premed student. I thought it would give me tools to go out and do something," he recalls. "But the longer I was in it, the more I thought it was like a trade school might be, if it taught you to do just that and nothing else. I wanted to go outside the box of that degree program and think more broadly."

Glenn took classes in literature, writing, and history, and all the philosophy courses he could with Harry Jellema, a towering figure whose students went on to head philosophy departments at prestigious schools including Duke, Notre Dame and Yale. One philosophical hot topic of the day particularly caught Glenn's interest. In a 1959 lecture at Cambridge University, British author and physicist Charles Percy Snow had described what he called "the two cultures," natural scientists and literary intellectuals. Snow contended that the gap between the two had grown dangerously wide, with each group ignorant and dismissive of the other's work.

Snow's assertion sparked spirited, international debate. But it struck Glenn as being right on the money. In his courses at Calvin, he experienced those two cultures. "There were the scientific types who dealt with analytic, microscopic, technical things but did not venture much beyond that. And there were the literary types who talked about wonderful things, had great ideas and sort of massaged each other but didn't really affect the world much." He didn't quite fit with the literary types, who deemed it a badge of honor to flunk the science courses that he aced. He didn't quite fit with the scientists, who stuck to equations and theorems; he loved to write essays, memoirs, travelogues.

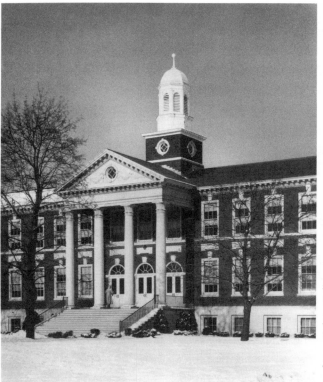

Archives, Calvin College

When Glenn attended Calvin College in the early 1960s, the white-pillared administration building was a campus landmark.

Within Calvin's vision of a true liberal arts education, Glenn found he could crisscross the two cultures, and for that, he loved the school. (In his sophomore year, when an alumni group gave him a $300 scholarship, he gave it all to a fundraising drive to build the college a new campus.) But for all Glenn learned at Calvin, as graduation neared, he felt its limitations.

Just as when he had paged through *National Geographic* as a boy, he felt drawn to another, wider world. "I knew there was something out there. The question was, are we content to stay inside? Because this hermetically sealed environment was pretty comfortable—nobody was wealthy, but nobody was poor; we were all well fed. I knew if I stayed in a place like that, I'd probably not have a new idea in my life, though I'd learn to recite the old ones very well. That did not feel reassuring to me."

A Calvin degree required 124 course hours, with major and minor subject-matter concentrations. In his final semester, Glenn was surpassing 250 hours. He showed administrators how he had met the requirements for two complete degrees: a bachelor's of arts with a major in English literature and philosophy and a minor in German, and a bachelor's of science with a major in biology and chemistry and a minor in history.

No, not quite, he was told. For each degree, physical education credit was required—and he had taken only one gym class. "Okay," he recalls thinking, "if they want to play bureaucrat, I can do that.'" He repeated the phys ed class, including a requirement that seemed taxing at the time: running a full mile.

He still has his Calvin assignment notebook, the red-leather binder embossed with the school emblem, shot through with dust from years in the attic. Scotch-taped inside its front cover are the now-yellowed sheets where he tracked due dates for papers. A handwritten schedule, headed "May-June" and covering several sheets of ruled paper, lists 135 things to be accomplished. Paper-clipped to a notebook divider is a memento from Blodgett: a cellophane-wrapped, curved suture needle threaded with a fine pale blue thread.

Affixed to the top of the notebook's first page is a quotation clipped from a newspaper. The quotation reads, "I am determined to finish, but not to incarcerate myself in the ridiculous medical profession. Those six or seven years lost in the study of a career are the most monstrous interest society exacts from its crooked leaders, because they coincide with the most beautiful years of our lives." Its attribution line reads, "Che Guevara, while a medical student."

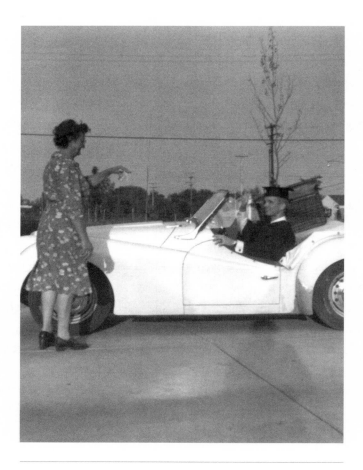

Glenn Geelhoed in his Calvin College graduation robes in 1964 with his mother Alice and the Triumph TR-3 sports car he bought with his earnings from jobs during college.

CHAPTER THREE

Imagination and Organization

HIS LAST MONTHS AT CALVIN COLLEGE FOUND GLENN FILLING OUT applications for medical schools—and, to keep his options open, for other graduate schools—while doing more than a little soul-searching. The glossy brochures and course catalogs from the medical schools were impressive, almost intimidating in the abundance of what they offered: state-of-the-art class and lab settings, eminent professors, accommodations that looked plush by Calvin standards. Browsing these rich settings, especially for graduate schools, began to feel like "eating dessert all day," he recalls. The more he read what the medical schools proposed to do for him, the more he pondered another question: What am I going to do that will do good for anyone else?

Doubting he could afford most of them, Glenn applied to seven medical schools, including the University of Chicago, Harvard, Northwestern and the University of Michigan. He never will forget the week the responses came: on Monday, two letters, both acceptances; on Tuesday and Wednesday, five more, all acceptances. With six of them, the tuition costs were staggering, even with scholarships and grants. In the letter from the University of Michigan Medical School, he found better news: the offer of a National Merit Scholarship that would pay his entire medical-school bill if he maintained a grade-point average of 3.75.

He decided where to travel for in-person interviews based on which medical schools he most wished to attend, but also which he could visit economically. His trip to the University of Chicago was memorable for one bizarre episode. The interviewing physician welcomed Glenn to his office, asked him to say a few words about himself, and then sat wordlessly, chain-smoking. Whenever Glenn stopped speaking, the physician waved for him to continue but said nothing. After about fifteen minutes of monologue, Glenn thanked the interviewer for his time. As he walked out of the office, a secretary intercepted him and asked him to wait. A moment later, the mute interviewer emerged, introduced himself as the chair of the psychiatry department, and explained the silent treatment was his way of gauging how applicants handled adversity and ambiguity. A+, he told Glenn. Thanks, Glenn said—but thought, *No thanks.*

On his visit to Harvard, Glenn took the subway from the Boston airport to save cab fare. Lugging a plaid suitcase up from the subway station into the snow, he walked among storied school landmarks: the imposing U-shaped cluster of the medical school buildings; the Peter Bent Brigham Hospital, with its classic pillared facade. He found a wing of classrooms open and stood in the back of one, thinking what it would be like to study there. But the next day, the interviews with medical-school administrators felt perfunctory, blasé—as if they were thinking, *Of course you want to come here. Everyone does.* The haughtiness and costliness of Harvard concerned Glenn as much as the excellence and prestige of the place attracted him.

At the University of Michigan, the equation shifted: Big opportunities and, after scholarships, little cost. At Michigan, Glenn felt the same tug he'd felt for years between the sciences and the humanities. He had applied for and been accepted to Michigan's medical school, where the National Merit Scholarship would pay his way; he also had applied to graduate school there, and for a Woodrow Wilson Fellowship that would largely cover grad-school costs. At the screening for the Wilson fellowship, interviewers quizzed Glenn about his intentions: *If you're accepted to both, how will you make up your mind?* He answered that he might use a technique recommended by Sigmund Freud: "When you have a difficult decision to make, you flip a coin, and when you are sorry that it came up heads, you have made your decision." The response seemed to amuse the screening committee, which offered him the fellowship.

Faced finally with deciding, Glenn didn't need the coin flip. If he enrolled in medical school now, he reasoned, he probably could go to graduate school later. But if he chose graduate school first, he might not get another chance at medical-school admission plus a scholarship to Michigan, one of the finest medical schools in the nation. His choice was clear.

At Calvin College, Glenn had been one of four thousand students. At U-M, he joined a student body of 52,000, and a medical school class of 240. It was a small school within a mega-university, the best of both worlds for him. Living on campus for the first time, he felt much more a part of everything, from the blue-and-gold school spirit to the heady '60s mix of music, politics and protests. In "the Diag" at the heart of campus, he reveled in chance meetings with students from all backgrounds and disciplines: artists, engineers, architects. With medical-school classmates who also were humanities buffs, he helped stage the play *Waiting for Godot* and a choral performance of Berlioz' *Requiem*. He founded a literary magazine named *The Paeon*—the name of the physician to Olympian gods and a pun on med students' lowly, peon status.

Glenn loved medical school from the start. Though classmates groaned at the enormous amount of material to be memorized, he felt certain he'd find some use for everything he learned. In classes where students jockeyed to score a tenth of a percent higher than the next guy, he strove hard for grades but resolved not to be as cutthroat as the hypercompetitive students known as "gunners."

Of the specialties, he especially liked studying endocrinology and neurology—and anatomy, partly because of the interest he had nursed since his fish-gutting days but also because of the company. Most days in anatomy lab, a blond-haired fellow student found some reason to come to his table. He was pretty sure she was flirting; he was quite sure he liked it.

Sally Ryden, raised in the comfortable suburbs east of Detroit, was also a National Merit Scholarship student. She was very bright and, he thought, beautiful in an offbeat way. Their medical textbooks called the heavy-lidded look of her right eye a ptosis, a congenital eyelid droop. He remembers thinking, *bedroom eyes.*

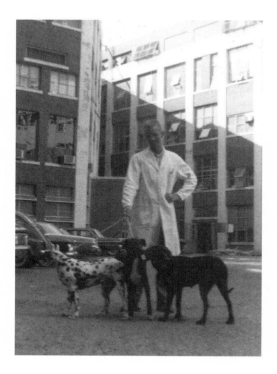

Glenn with lab animals on which he operated during medical school at the University of Michigan.

Another of Sally's distinguishing traits: She was an ace at studying and learning in traditional, by-the-book ways. Glenn, by contrast, was more the experiential learner, hitting the books but also scavenging and absorbing knowledge from all around him. "We are totally different people," Sally once told him. "I take multiple-choice exams; you write essays."

What Sally called differences, Glenn saw more as ways they complemented and dovetailed with each other. By early 1965, they were discussing how to balance med school and marriage. But a wedding ceremony would have to wait until Glenn's return from his first trip abroad—the kind of adventure he had imagined since childhood.

In July 1965, Glenn got off a Pan American Clipper airship in Santo Domingo, the Dominican Republic, with no visa in his pocket, only a few Spanish words in his head, and a copy of a UN document authorizing his entry into the country to provide emergency medical assistance. Subma-chine-gun-toting soldiers escorted him to the baggage claim; a U.S. embassy official met him there and then drove him across the island, passing through police checkpoints by waving the UN papers.

Since the early 1930s, the island nation had been run by Rafael Trujillo, a dictator whose brutality the United States overlooked because he was staunchly anticommunist. After Trujillo's assassination in 1961, reformist and military factions wrestled for control of the government. In April 1965, after months of dark warnings about "communist danger" and "another Cuba," then-President Lyndon Johnson ordered 22,000 troops to the island. During the occupation by the 82nd Airborne, factional fighting ended and a U.S.–friendly government was installed—and a dysentery epidemic struck the impoverished, desperate population.

When a World Health Organization–sponsored medical mission to the Dominican Republic recruited volunteers at the University of Michigan, Glenn had jumped at the chance to join. As the embassy driver navigated roads pocked from shelling, Glenn soaked in his first views of a tropical para-dise turned armed camp: military helicopters hovering beyond the waving palm trees, U.S. battleships lined up beyond the blue surf crashing on silver beaches. Naked Dominican kids scampered around the sandbagged installa-tions built for recoilless rifles.

Glenn had arranged to stay in the home of an evacuated missionary fam-ily for eight weeks while working at clinics to diagnose, treat and rehydrate patients—many of them children—who otherwise might not survive dys-entery. Reporting to one of the island's main hospitals to begin work, he was shocked to find the 180-bed facility had no running water or refrigeration and only minimal staff and supplies, not even aspirin. There were no laboratory instruments to measure electrolytes, to establish what kind of dehydration a child had; no way to culture specimens to learn what organisms were caus-ing illnesses; not even a scale, leaving practitioners to guess children's weight in dispensing treatment. "Even if we had a diagnosis, we couldn't be sure of getting the antibiotic of choice to treat it with," Glenn wrote in his trip notes.

The medical teams kept reporting to work, improvising and stretching every precious shipment of donated supplies. But as Dominican factions continued to skirmish, the volunteers were caught in the middle. Glenn's journal records the day when a general of one faction, "down to only his air force and a radio station, gamely went on the air and announced 'Operation Cleanup,' declaring the precise rebel areas that his air force was going to strafe and rocket and urging the people to leave these areas. His announced targets were the bridge we passed over in entering the city, the large fortress close to the district where I stayed, and the heavily populated area around the rebel radio station. The rebel radio promptly, screamed, 'Into the streets, patriots! Do not leave! If you die, you die for liberty!'"

In the hours before U.S. Marines arrived and the strafing stopped, many Dominicans were killed in the streets or in their homes, Glenn wrote. At a house in the U.S. embassy compound where he and other civilians had taken shelter, he watched the assault from a rooftop deck. "During the strafing," he wrote, "the American children would run to one side of the house and watch the planes work on the bridge, then run to the other side and watch them riddle the neighborhood of the radio station."

That night, U.S.-passport-holding civilians were to be evacuated, ferried by Marine Corps helicopters to the U.S.S. *Boxer* aircraft carrier sitting just offshore. Glenn was left with a choice: wave his UN papers and remain on the island as an "international citizen" or claim his U.S. citizenship and be airlifted to the *Boxer*. He hated to leave, as the clinic work had just begun going well, but he knew medical supplies were running low at the rehydration sites.

With all the mobile military might on the island, he reasoned, there must be a way to put it to good use. "I figured, why not shoot the moon?" On the first of what would be many global medical adventures, Glenn took an approach that would become his trademark: He colored outside the lines.

While on the mission, Glenn had kept in touch with Sally via ham radio. Sally and her family had licenses and radios, and so did the missionaries whose home Glenn was using. As Americans in the embassy compound prepared to be evacuated, Glenn talked his way past guards at the compound gate and raced back to the missionaries' home. Jotting lists of the medical supplies the clinics needed, he fired up the radio. He got a call through to

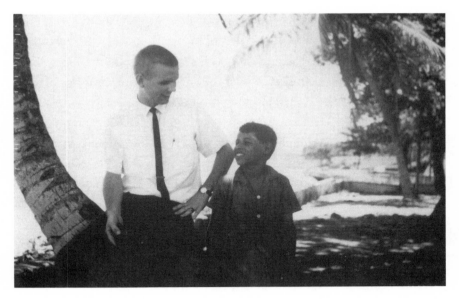

On his first foreign medical mission trip to the Dominican Republic, Glenn made friends with Santo Domingo's children.

Georgia-based Medical Assistance Programs (MAP International), a charity that supplies medical and disaster relief supplies, and asked for as much as the group could send. Then he recruited Sally and family to help him patch radio contacts from the island through to telephones in the United States.

On board the *Boxer*, he chatted up the service personnel and medics. "Would you like me to get a message to your folks?" he asked. Sure, many answered. With Sally as operator, Glenn helped one serviceman reach his mom in Idaho and another reach a sweetheart in Arkansas. When the grateful troops asked what they could do to thank him, Glenn's answer was instant and brassy: How about IV kits, vitamins, nutrient bars, as much as you've got? How about a loan of army trucks to get supplies out to the clinics? Describing the adventure later to Sally, Glenn observed, "It's amazing what you can do with a little bit of imagination and organization."

Fourteen days later, Glenn was on the beach as a huge shipment of supplies arrived from MAP and other U.S. charities: fluids, antibiotics, vitamins— thirty-six tons in all. This time, the military-style maneuver Glenn witnessed was a joyful one: two hulking landing crafts plowing onto the Dominican beach and disgorging pallet after pallet of medical supplies. The volunteers worked round-the-clock the next four weeks to get supplies to patients and practitioners who needed them. When they needed more hands to sort and label the supplies, they bribed local boys to help by promising them an irresistible reward: a baseball game umpired by the *americanos*, in Santo Domingo's deserted national stadium, where cows grazed in the outfield.

From Glenn's last day on the island, his journal recounts a visit to a barrio so poor that residents lived in shacks fashioned from banana leaves. When Glenn and a colleague arrived with cases of vitamins, "a curious crowd quickly gathered, and we lined them up with the high ideals of instructing them to take only one bottle and only one of the pills each day," he wrote. But latecomers surged forward, fearing they'd miss the giveaway; they rushed the two Americans, swarming and rocking their car.

Glenn dropped a carton, pill bottles scattered, and as residents fought to snatch them, the two men struggled to the car and sped away. The episode was "a failure as personal diplomacy," Glenn wrote, "but it was a lesson in the magnitude of the problems that confront charitable intentions."

Despite setbacks, Glenn didn't feel overwhelmed by the challenges on the island, he said later, because he figured any contribution he could make would be an improvement. Over decades of similar experiences in bleak, deprived environments, Glenn would refine this observation into a full-blown philosophy. Like most of his philosophical conclusions, he has thought it through until he can state it exactly as he means it—and, for good measure, in both a short, aphoristic version and a longer, more explanatory one.

The short version of his philosophy on serving in impoverished settings is, "You can't fall off the floor." And the longer one: "When you're in a failed state, your job isn't to make it look like where you came from. Your job is simply to stave off entropic collapse for one more day—to do whatever you can to make changes for the better."

His boyish looks earned Glenn a nickname among some Dominicans: *americanito*, the little American guy. But in his time on the island, he also earned a big reputation. An article about the mission trip, in a 1966 medical

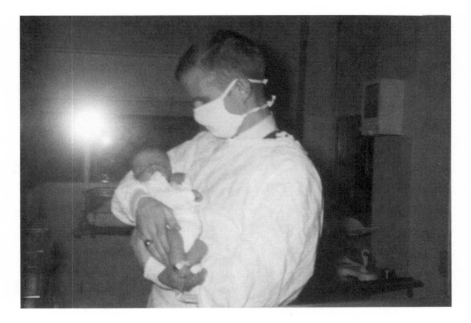

Glenn holds his son Donald William Geelhoed, born on March 9, 1966.

society journal, reported that Glenn was "known as the *americanito* who could be counted on to help when others couldn't."

Two weeks after Glenn left the Dominican Republic, he and Sally stood at the altar of the Ann Arbor Christian Reformed Church and exchanged vows before their closest relatives and friends. The honeymoon was the long weekend they could grab before returning to medical-school classes.

Through their demanding second-year coursework, the two Geelhoeds ran neck and neck on grades. After three grueling days of exams that capped the spring semester, both felt they had done well. So the next day they slept in—until the pregnant Sally rolled over and her husband felt something soak the bed sheets. An hour and a half after Sally's water broke, on March 9, 1966, the couple welcomed a son: Donald William Geelhoed, with a middle name honoring his grandfather and a first name memorializing Glenn's onetime classmate Donald Gabrielson.

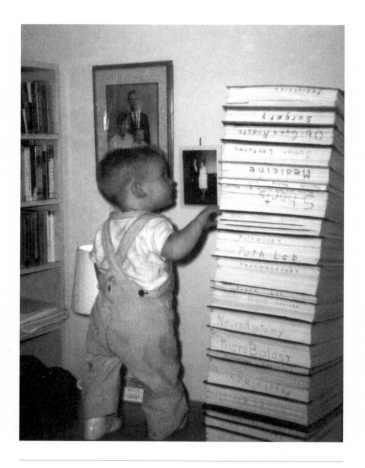

In the Geelhoed home, both parents in medical school meant stacks of books and notes taller than toddler Donald.

CHAPTER FOUR

Beyond "Medical Center Civilization"

PERHAPS THE TRAIT CAME PARTLY FROM HIS FATHER, WILLIAM, WHO
was masterful at remembering significant dates. Perhaps it came partly from his
mother, Alice, who delighted in baking for special occasions. Whatever its ori-
gins, Glenn Geelhoed's fixation is clear: He's devoutly observant of birthdays.

He situates other events in time by noting their proximity to loved ones'
birthdays. He insists on merry birthday rituals such as letting honorees choose
any food to be served on their special day—even the most nutritionally bank-
rupt, despite his devotion to healthful eating. Mindful of how quickly children's lives seem to pass, he makes a ritual of celebrating half birthdays as well
as actual birth dates.

So it pleases him to recall that the young Geelhoed family's first medical
mission began on his twenty-sixth birthday and encompassed Donald's second. The chubby, tow-headed boy turned two surrounded by youngsters who
could not have looked less like him—in Nigeria.

In 1967, the young couple's hectic life was captured in what is still one of
Glenn's favorite snapshots: a diaper-wearing Donald standing next to a stack
of his parents' medical-school study notes that is taller than he is. Despite the
competing demands of parenting and coursework, both Geelhoeds were stellar
students. In the next-to-last semester of their senior year, when U of M medical

students were encouraged to arrange off-campus clinical experiences, Sally and Glenn's first choice was a foreign fellowship program run by the Association of American Medical Colleges.

They made an enticing pitch: two Doctors Geelhoed for the price of one. They were awarded a grant to spend three months working in east-central Nigeria at Takum Christian Hospital, the only medical center in a vast, needy district. While they prepared for the trip, civil war broke out as Nigeria tried to reclaim the breakaway region that had declared its independence as Biafra.

For a time the U.S. state department warned the Geelhoeds it might not approve travel to an area deemed so dangerous. Finally they were cleared to go, and on January 19, 1968, Glenn's birthday gift was a bumpy but intact landing on the Takum airstrip.

An hour after they arrived, the Geelhoeds were making hospital rounds with the Stehouwers: Dr. Ed and his wife, Dr. Flora, the only physicians on staff. The crash course in the pace of bush medicine began before the Geelhoeds even entered the wards, as two patients were brought in needing emergency

The Geelhoed family is greeted on the landing strip at Takum Christian Hospital in east-central Nigeria. During their senior year of medical school, Sally and Glenn spent three months working at the hospital, the only medical center serving a vast area of the impoverished nation.

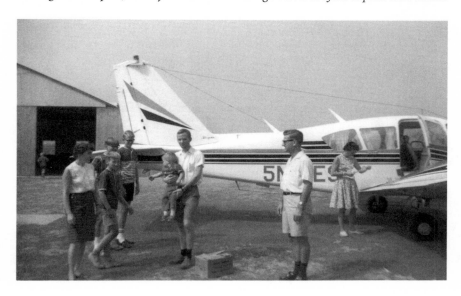

hernia repairs. While the Geelhoeds assisted with the operations, Donald toddled around his new environment. Glenn remembers a Nigerian tyke checking under Donald's diaper to see if the newcomer really was white all over.

Supported by mission sponsors including the Christian Reformed Church, Takum Christian Hospital was officially a 140-bed facility. But as Glenn noted in his journals from the trip, "Just how many patients are hospitalized at any given time is only approximated by the number of beds . . . The ward designations for some patients may be 'bed 18' and 'bed 18-½,' the '½' representing the floor-mat space between beds."

Despite the hospital's strained resources, Glenn saw it delivering "amazingly good-quality care," treating many patients quickly and serviceably without what he called "the frills of university technique." He praised the native nurses who so ably screened and cared for patients that only the sickest 10 percent had to be referred to doctors (and who did double duty as translators between the local Hausa dialect and English, the nation's official language). Glenn also found local practitioners' approach to death admirably down-to-earth. "Everyone in this primitive society is intimately acquainted with death," he wrote, "and since death is such a common experience, it does not require the presence of an observer entitled with an MD to pronounce it."

In the United States, both Geelhoeds had received superb training in what Glenn called "medical center civilization." But what they encountered in Nigeria would forever alter Glenn's understanding of medicine, and of his calling in it.

The wards of Takum threw the whole world's health problems into sharp relief. In the developed world, parasitic diseases were seldom grave or life-threatening; in the developed world, infectious diseases had become "the great showcase of modern medicine in which civilization displays the control achieved over disease," Glenn wrote. But the same diseases "cannot be subdued" in the developing world, he noted, for lack of so much else: sanitation systems and clean water, safe and sufficient food and shelter, health care and hygiene education, transportation to treatment.

One example: Among patients at Takum, a filarial worm parasite spread by biting flies was "almost universal," Glenn reported. Its infestations caused gross swellings, deep muscle abscesses, and a progressive loss of vision commonly called "river blindness." The only available treatment was hazardous and uncomfortable—and if patients survived the treatment and were cured, they would go home to the same swarming flies and almost certain re-infestation.

What he observed hit Glenn hard and cemented two convictions: that the world's health problems defied simple fixes, and that where solutions could be found, he wanted to help find them.

Every day in Takum taught the Geelhoeds something new and challenged their assumptions. Seeing parents struggle to feed and house the children they already had, "we first presumed that we would be treating many women with demands for birth-control assistance," Glenn wrote in his journal. "Much to our surprise, the reverse was true: had not limits been placed on such use of the physician's time, it would have been too easy to become involved in running a full-time infertility clinic. The greatest sociologic and economic disgrace among the natives was to be barren."

Most of the girls in the area, he learned, were married as soon as they hit child-bearing age, at a standard bride price that was about half of what locals could fetch for a prize cow. From the time the brides were bought until menopause or death, they were expected to produce a child every other year—a tradition that had existed as long as anyone could remember. "To insure survival of a few children, a dozen births were once mandatory," Glenn noted. "Now, half of these babies can be expected to mature." But the social imperative remained to keep bearing them, even as the exploding population strained village resources to the breaking point.

To his journal, he confessed "a twinge of guilt" when performing procedures "designed to restore fertility to patients in whom we thought contraceptive measures were better indicated." But the underlying lesson was one he would never forget, and would later share with countless others: that what "Doctor knows best" from one culture might have little relevance in another.

Coming to Nigeria meant Sally and Glenn would miss the climactic event of the medical-school experience: the ritual known as match day. Like their med-school colleagues, both had completed the steps of the match process. They had interviewed at hospitals where they might want to spend the next

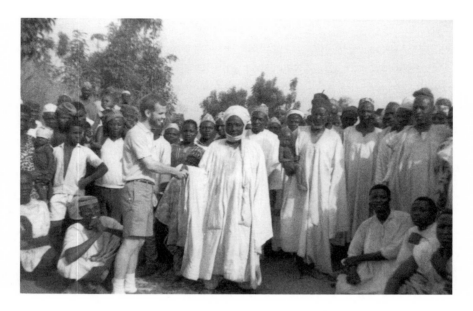

Glenn meets the chiefs whose clanspeople came to Takum Christian Hospital for care. His first medical mission experience in Africa convinced Glenn that "amazingly good quality care" could be provided even in humble settings.

few years as residents, getting specialty training. They had listed the institutions where they would most like to serve residencies. And they had submitted those lists to the binding match system, devoutly hoping that the institutions they ranked high would also list them as top-ranked choices.

Sally's chosen specialty was pathology; she was very good at looking at a slide or specimen and recognizing the clinical and anatomic patterns that led to a diagnosis. Since his college days moonlighting at the hospital, Glenn had appreciated the immediacy of surgical relief of patient problems and had thought that being a surgeon might suit his temperament and skills. The Nigeria experience convinced him of that absolutely.

An article Glenn later wrote about the trip, for a medical-student journal, included an exquisite understatement: "Surgery is not without its problems under primitive conditions." One example he encountered involved securing blood for transfusions. It meant convincing villagers that donating would not drain out their life spirit, as many believed. But even where a host of factors were beyond his control, Glenn found he often could effect "immediate, definitive cures" with little more than a scalpel and sutures.

From living with scarce water supply under a baking tropical sun, scores of patients arrived each week with hideous, infected skin ulcers that could lead to blood poisoning, deformity and even death. Almost as numerous were the patients with severe burns: toddlers who tumbled into cooking fires, children caught when winds shifted the bush fires set to clear the savannah grass. And then there were the epileptics, many brought in after their severely burned limbs were contracting and deformed by scarring. Explanations of how they'd fallen into fires during seizures never entirely dispelled suspicions that they'd been exposed to flames to "drive out demons." Still, in all but the gravest cases, Glenn could effectively treat these patients with a relatively minor operations and skin grafts.

If surgery was not a silver bullet, it was at least, as he once wrote, "a particularly gratifying mode of health care." He could operate to deliver infants whose teenaged mothers were too small to give birth naturally; he could operate to retrieve stillborn infants and repair shattered wombs after women labored too long in the bush. With relatively quick, contained acts, he could significantly restore health. And he could achieve that without everything Takum didn't have—might never have—to manage medical conditions: technology, transportation, sanitation, education.

In his medical journal article about the trip, Glenn ranked surgery on a par with antibiotics "as the most successful form of medicine that can be practiced" in the resource-poor, developing world.

Beyond the operating room, some of the Geelhoeds' most interesting experiences came on treks to outlying villages for preventive-medicine missions. News that the doctors were coming was passed first by shortwave radio, then out to the most remote villages by the sonorous signals of native drums. By the time the medical team arrived, long lines of the sick had formed, and large crowds of the curious.

While local mothers jockeyed for a chance to cuddle Donald, his parents examined patients, dispensed treatment, gave hygiene lectures and administered vaccines: tetanus, smallpox, whooping cough, measles—diseases well controlled in the developed world, but potentially lethal in these villages. As a bonus of the public health forays, Glenn noted in his journal, "we often returned with gifts from the patients we had treated—a few yams from some families, a bull's horn from another, and usually a loudly squawking rooster.

"I always felt as uncomfortable as the chicken when this disgruntled gift was presented," he wrote, "since we knew that this was a significant gift which might have been a whole family's protein intake for a month. But there was no refusing their hospitality, because they were too elated that the threat of measles and tetanus was lifted from their hut to worry about malnutrition."

After one visit to a remote outpost, the Geelhoeds were heading back to Takum in a Peugeot station wagon driven by hospital colleague Flora Stehouwer. Though Flora had logged hours driving on the district's baked-mud roads, that day the steering got away from her. A wheel careened off a rut in the road, and the Peugeot began to flip. Glenn, in the front seat, had time only to reach around and push Donald to the floorboard as the car tumbled onto the driver's side and skidded across the dirt, engulfed in a cloud of dust.

Glenn was banged up but able to crawl from the car. Though blinded by the dust, he could hear Donald's terrified crying and pulled the toddler out first. Next he retrieved Sally, limp and unconscious, and placed her in the shade of a tree with Donald. Flora was slumped over the crushed steering wheel, but she awakened as Glenn sought to pry her out. She was able to hobble from the car and join Donald, still squalling, and Sally, conscious but in too much pain to move. Bleeding from cut knees, Glenn did the only thing he could think of to get help: He picked up Donald and began walking up the road toward Takum, some twenty-five kilometers away.

Village children gaped as the white man limped by, a toddler on his hip and blood trickling down his legs. Spying a man with a bicycle, Glenn summoned enough local dialect to explain about the crash and beg the man to carry a message to Takum Christian Hospital, to send help. The man said he'd be glad to, for a price: local currency worth roughly five dollars. Furious at the grasping request but with no money on him, Glenn convinced the man to take a promissory note—a page from his ever-present notepad on which he scrawled an I.O.U. with the addendum, "YOU BASTARD."

An hour later, a cargo truck appeared, and Glenn flagged it down and again explained about the accident. The driver invited him and Donald in and drove them back to the crash site. Glenn checked on Flora and Sally, who both were in pain but holding up. While Glenn did that, the driver used a length of hose to siphon gas from the wrecked Peugeot into his truck, and then drove off alone, without looking back.

Glenn set out again with Donald, but after another hour, he saw, in the distance, a dust cloud on the road that seemed to be drawing nearer. The bicyclist had earned his payment after all. After he had delivered Glenn's message, Takum Christian dispatched all of its three vehicles, each carrying stretchers, IV bottles, other medical equipment and personnel.

Flora had a minor lung laceration from a broken rib but recovered swiftly. Sally fared less well. Her pelvis was broken, which meant considerable pain and strict bed rest for most of the rest of the fellowship.

With Sally laid up, Glenn worked even longer hours. But every part of the experience fascinated him, and he filled notebooks writing about it, recording every detail he thought might help him later reflect on events and extract meaning from them. From those notes, he drew the conclusion of his medical journal article: "The exposure to world health problems that this fellowship afforded has great shock value," he wrote. "The fellowship placed in perspective the narrow world of esoteric medical care in the health centers of civilization by showing us the other side of the twentieth-century world-health enigma: population masses dying of disease that can be simply controlled."

His final statement about the trip left no doubt that it would not be his last: "It was the high point of our clinical education, and an experience enjoyable enough to be contagious."

In one of his most vivid memories from the trip, Glenn is walking to the hospital one morning when a nearly naked, barefoot boy approaches, signaling that he has something to deliver. He gives Glenn an envelope, wrinkled and soiled from passage through many hands. Weeks after most of their fellow students received their residency match letters, the Geelhoeds' letter has found them in dusty, dirt-poor Takum. The news is all they had hoped for: residencies for Sally in pathology and Glenn in surgery at Harvard Medical School.

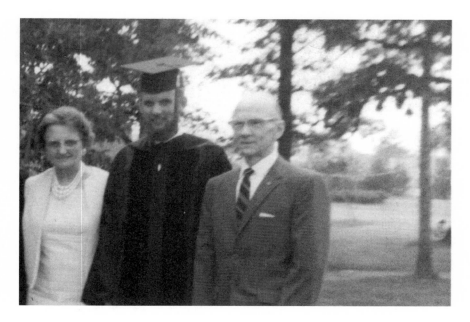

Glenn with his parents at the commencement ceremonies for the University of Michigan Medical School's Class of 1968.

At the commencement ceremonies for the University of Michigan Medical School's class of 1968, the Geelhoeds graduated at the top of their class—Sally first. Donald sat with the throng of relatives who came to watch the first Doctors Geelhoed receive their diplomas. Like many of their fellow grads, Glenn and Sally wore peace-sign pendants with their robes, in solidarity with the movements on their campus and others against the Vietnam War.

The week after the commencement, Bill Geelhoed retired from Kindel. His three daughters, all teachers, had completed their master's degrees; Glenn was now "my son the doctor." The man who had so longed to graduate college himself had seen all of his children do so with distinction and press on to advanced degrees. He could not have been more proud.

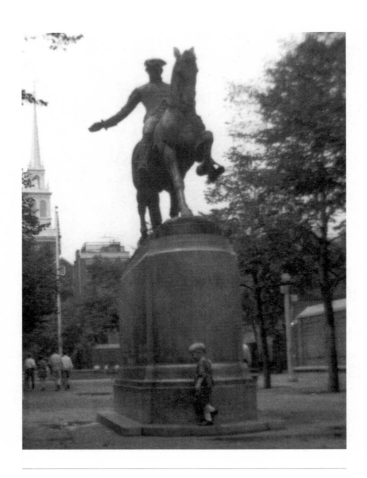

Donald Geelhoed in front of a statue of Paul Revere near Boston's Old North Church, August, 1969.

CHAPTER FIVE

"Just Keep Operating and Learning"

THE 1960 FORD GALAXIE HARDTOP WAS SO RIDDLED WITH RUST THAT its gas tank had to be braced inside the chassis with two-by-fours and copper wire, lest it fall off in transit. After a rousing send-off from Glenn's relatives in west Michigan, the Geelhoeds nursed the old car eastbound on hope and 21-cents-a-gallon gas. Destination: Boston, Massachusetts, and the teaching hospitals of Harvard.

In 1911, a hospital "for the care of sick persons in indigent circumstances" was established with a bequest from a Boston real estate baron and restaurateur named Peter Bent Brigham. By the late 1960s the hospital, known familiarly as "the Brigham," was a landmark among the Harvard Medical School buildings along Huntington Avenue, and a hub of learning for Harvard medical residents.

Sally Geelhoed would serve her pathology residency at the Brigham. Surgical resident Glenn Geelhoed would spend his first year rotating through services there, studying anesthesiology, orthopedics and other specialties as well as general surgery. Donald, big and verbal for his age, would be in daycare near the Brigham, with his parents tag-teaming pickups and drop-offs depending on their shifts. Home was a two-bedroom apartment in nearby

Brookline, a block from John F. Kennedy's birthplace. The young doctors' duties were to begin on July 1, 1968. So to get their bearings and set up house-keeping they arrived in town the second week of June.

At the Brigham, first-year surgery residents were given a title borrowed from the British medical system: house officer. The title was meant to confer status—a cut above, the chosen ones. But in practice, being a house officer chiefly meant working long, unpredictable hours to the point of exhaustion. In a journal entry, Glenn improvised rules for surviving the assignment: "When standing, look for a place to sit. When sitting, look for a place to lie. The dinner you have had they cannot take away from you. Just keep operating and learning, no matter the hours."

But if residents could stand the pace, they'd have a chance to study with giants of the field—eminent, internationally known physicians who most medical students knew only as names in textbooks: Dr. Joseph E. Murray, whose team was the first to successfully transplant kidneys from both cadavers and live donors, and whose work earned him the Nobel Prize; Dr. Frances D. Moore—called "Franny" behind his back but never to his face—the Brigham surgeon-in-chief as admired for his professional prowess as he was feared for his iron-fisted leadership.

Though Glenn wasn't due to start for more than two weeks, he decided to drop by the hospital to say hello upon arrival in Boston. The orientation pamphlet had warned that "No vacation time is scheduled into the surgical house officer's year, but if the incoming group of house officers can be convinced to start early," the departing group might grab a vacation break. As Glenn remembers it, he had barely set foot on the surgical wing "when someone sang out, 'New house officer's here!'—and then all I saw were the backs of others scurrying out."

Administrators told Glenn where to pick up his white coat and pager. Too excited about the new assignment to object, he just smiled and complied. He had pocketed the pager and was on his way to get the coat when the pager went off, telling him to report to the operating room. He would be assisting as legendary surgeon Moore completed a liver transplant—only the second to be performed at the Brigham—in a sixteen-year-old boy named Tommy.

Organ transplantation was still very much a new frontier, regarded with awe by some and with pessimism by others. Though liver transplants in humans had been attempted since the early '60s, the patients did not survive long, typically because their bodies' immune systems rejected the new organ. The first successful human liver transplant—in which the patient lived another thirteen months—had occurred just months before Glenn found himself scrubbing in to Franny Moore's operating room.

A tumor in Tommy's liver was so large that removing the entire organ offered the only hope of cure. At the nearby Children's Hospital Boston, a trauma victim had been declared brain dead and permission had been obtained for organ donation. The transplant team would be led by Moore and Dr. Alan Birtch, a junior staff surgeon at the Brigham who had been a surgical resident himself only a few years before. Because the transplant process was essentially three operations in one—harvesting the donated liver, removing the diseased liver, and suturing the donated organ in its place—it would take a team of doctors, nurses and support staff, and eight to ten hours to complete, even if all went well.

After brief introductions between team members and the new house officer, Glenn was gowned and gloved. His task as surgical assistant was to "hold the hooks," the surgical retractors on either side of the two-foot-long incision that opened Tommy's rib cage and gave Birtch and Moore room to work. As the hours passed, nurses and anesthesiologists could come and go, though few on the team left after they were spelled, eager to witness the event. As soon as one step of the operation was completed, the next began, smoothly and without fanfare. Glenn remembers marveling that even in the intense, high-stakes circumstances there was a palpable sense of camaraderie. When the transplant operation was completed and Tommy wheeled off to recover, Glenn felt exhausted but exhilarated.

Assigned to monitor Tommy under the watchful direction of Birtch, Glenn virtually lived in the Brigham's intensive care unit. Though house officers ostensibly could grab naps in an on-call room furnished with bunks, it was far down the corridor (called "the Brigham Pike") from Tommy's room. The only closer break room was the Cutler Lounge, outside the Brigham's operating suite. Wallpapered with sailing charts of the waters around Cape Cod, the lounge reeked of tobacco smoke, as did the old red leather couch along one wall. When Glenn asked one of the nurses where he might nap, she pointed to the couch with the joking reassurance, "Don't worry—it will never be for more than an hour."

As Glenn watched, Tommy's new liver functioned beautifully while everything else shut down. The boy was awake much of the time, and when he was feeling more healthy and hopeful, he would talk about returning to school. But the medications Tommy took to prevent rejection of the new liver impaired his body's ability to meet other challenges. When Tommy ran a persistent fever and blood cultures showed a bacterial infection, he was put on antibiotics. But as Glenn reviewed scores of repeat blood tests, it was clear the drugs weren't working. Bedridden and weakening, Tommy was put on a ventilator as his lungs began to fail.

On the forty-fifth day after the operation, Glenn was helping Birtch check Tommy's status. Glenn had his finger on Tommy's pulse and his eyes on an electrocardiogram monitor when Tommy's heart stopped. Glenn administered CPR but could not get the heart to rally. Still delivering compressions to Tommy's chest, Glenn looked up at Birtch, who nodded and turned away. Glenn turned off the heart monitors and noted the time of death on Tommy's chart. So far in his study of medicine, some lessons had been hard; this one was heartbreaking.

A few days later, as was customary, all of the practitioners involved in Tommy's care—from the consulting specialists and transplant surgeons to the nurses and residents – assembled to review and learn from his case. The setting was Brigham Levine Auditorium, an imposing hall where oil portraits of Harvard Medical School legends lined the walls. By unbreakable tradition at these review sessions, the auditorium's front-row chairs were reserved for the most eminent faculty physicians. Junior medical staff could sit behind them, with visitors and guests seated next, and residents and medical students filling the back rows.

Birtch ran the conference, calling on each practitioner in turn to contribute his or her data and analysis. A gastroenterology specialist noted that

Tommy died with a normal bilirubin reading, meaning the liver was working to the last. An infectious disease specialist discussed the 347 cultures that diagnosed the infection, and the antibiotics regimen that could not conquer it.

Moore, who at that time was writing a book on transplantation, laid out his vision for the future of transplantation and how grim outcomes such as Tommy's nonetheless helped move the science forward. Then, typical as it was for Moore to have the last word at these events, he chose not to. He turned to the rows of residents and, as Glenn remembers it, said roughly this: "Dr. Geelhoed was this patient's primary-caring physician. Would he like to add any comments in summation?"

As he rose to speak, Glenn remembers feeling relief that he'd worn a necktie that day. He took his place at the podium, behind which loomed the stern-faced portrait of legendary Brigham professor Harvey Cushing, considered the father of neurosurgery.

Glenn's remarks took no more than three minutes. He introduced himself: recently returned from a medical mission to Nigeria, beginning his Brigham residency with Tommy as his first patient. Since other speakers had covered all the clinical details of the case, he wished to add only one more piece of information, not from the patient's medical records but from his billing records: "Tommy's hospitalization for forty-five days in the Brigham cost the sum of the health and welfare budget of the Federal Republic of Nigeria, a nation of 68 million souls."

Scanning the audience, he tried to read faces for reactions. In the front row, several looked dismissive; further back, startled or incredulous. For a long moment his statement hung in the air—clearly not popular, but also not challenged—until the conference adjourned. All the front-row physicians made brisk exits, except for one. He approached Glenn, looked into his eyes, and said four words: "You know, you're right." With that, Dr. Joe Murray, who would become one of the great mentors and inspirations of Glenn's life, went about his rounds.

At Harvard, faculty who taught Glenn and residents who served with him were struck by two things: his promise as a physician and his penchant for flouting conventions he deemed too confining. As they worked together on the liver transplant and other cases, Birtch formed this impression of Glenn: "He was extremely bright and very enthusiastic, and it appeared he was marching to a slightly different drummer."

Throughout his medical training, Glenn had dutifully learned every by-the-book technique and procedure that was required. But he had no qualms about setting prescribed approaches aside if he thought something else would work better, to serve patients or advance science.

During the mission in Nigeria, Glenn and an unschooled Nigerian colleague did so many hernia-repair operations that he lost count. So when he was assigned to perform one during his first months at Brigham, he thought he had it made. Watching Glenn's swift, consistent technique during the operation, supervising surgeon Dr. Richard Wilson quizzed him: "Where did you learn to do that?" Glenn answered lightly that he had "just fixed something like 186 hernias in Africa." Wilson's genial but barbed response: "Imagine that, 186 hernia repairs and every one of them wrong."

Little as he enjoyed the critique, Glenn appreciated what he learned from Wilson: that these early stage patients needed an approach that was slower, more careful than the one he had used with Nigeria's more advanced disease cases. But later, when he replayed the episode with fellow resident Alden Harken, Glenn's own yardstick for success became clear: A surgery professor may have sneered at his work, but the 186 patients didn't.

From their first conversations, often mumbled in middle-of-the-night handoffs of patients in their care, Glenn hit it off with Alden, who was a year ahead of him in the surgical-residency program. On one level, the two were very different. Alden's childhood in upper-crust New England bore little resemblance to Glenn's in woodsy west Michigan. But beyond that, they had much in common. Like Glenn, Alden had married a medical-school classmate, Laurel, who was now a Harvard resident in pediatrics. Like Glenn and Sally, Alden and Laurel were juggling medical training and parenthood. They were second-year residents when their first son, Dwight, was born. The Geelhoeds were second-year residents when a younger brother arrived for Donald, Michael Alan, born October 3, 1969.

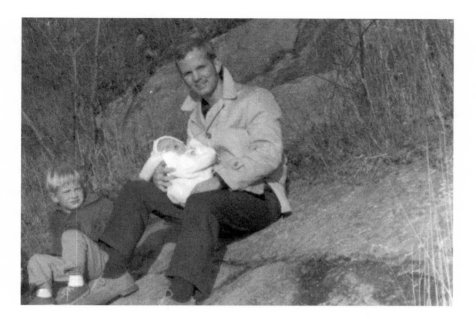

Glenn shared his love of the outdoors with his sons from their earliest days. Michael was only a few weeks old in November 1969 when Glenn—armed with his self-timer camera—took Michael and three-year-old Donald hiking on New Hampshire's Mount Monadnock.

Without his eyeglasses on, Alden could not see objects right in front of him. But as a learner, he sought constantly to broaden his vision, whether by reading the classics or by shadowing master surgeons in the operating room. When Glenn grumbled about being up late or rising early to study, he'd often find that Alden had matched him—or been up even later, or risen even earlier. To describe the two of them, Alden coined a teasing comparison: "I am not as smart as Glenn is, but I make up much of the difference in enthusiasm!"

Though he considered Glenn the more adventurous of the two of them, Alden had his moments. Once, after a black-tie medical-society dinner, strolling on one bank of the Charles River and looking toward the Massachusetts Institute of Technology on the other, Alden wondered aloud, "How far do you think it is from here to the other bank?" At the cost of a dry-cleaning tab (and a tuxedo that was never quite the same), he learned not just how far it was, but also how long it took to swim it.

Among Harvard medical educators and students, Glenn met plenty who, by Calvin College standards, would be deemed "prideful," people who expected to be recognized for their credentials, titles and pedigrees. In this crowd, Alden stood out—and impressed Glenn deeply—for his disarming lack of ego.

Glenn remembers the two of them standing among a group of Harvard medical students in the Bartlett Unit as they were preparing to walk rounds. "Alden is standing there with me, and next to us is Starling, the grandson of the great physiologist who had authored my physiology textbook. Next to him is Landis, whose father had broken new ground in the understanding of the heart. Next to him is Drinker, son of the inventor of the iron lung machine for artificial respiration. And next to him was the medical student assigned to me, Crichton"—Michael Crichton, whose first best-seller, *The Andromeda Strain*, was published while he was still in medical school, and who went on to fame for his science- and medical-themed movies (including *Jurassic Park*) and TV show (*ER*).

"And then there's Alden and me. And I looked around and said to him, 'Alden, everybody here is a big name except for you and me.' And Alden didn't get it. That's how unaffected he was; he didn't get the joke." Dr. Dwight Harken, Alden's father, is widely acknowledged as the father of heart surgery. He boasted a string of medical firsts, including being the first to develop and implant a heart pacemaker and the first to implant artificial heart valves (one of which bears his name). He also was the originator of hospital intensive care units to manage critically ill patients. But for all that, Alden—to Glenn's great delight—didn't get that the "big name" joke was on him.

The second year of residency was a uniquely privileged one for Glenn. Dr. Robert E. Gross, founder of both pediatric and cardiac surgery in the Harvard hospitals, was about to retire, and Glenn would be among the last residents to study pediatric surgery with him.

As a young surgeon at Children's Hospital Boston in the late-1930s, Gross earned his spurs by being a bit of a rebel. In autopsies of children who died of heart failure, he saw blood vessels that had failed to close normally after birth, a defect he believed he could repair with a relatively simple operation. His chief of surgery had misgivings, so Gross waited until his superior was out of town and got the acting chief's approval to try the operation. Later, Gross would note wryly that if the operation had not succeeded, he might have ended up a farmer. But it did succeed, and with one stroke he established his reputation as an innovator in both cardiac and pediatric surgery.

In the surgical suite where he taught Glenn and other residents, Gross had posted a sign that read, "If an operation is difficult, you are not doing it correctly." He knew precisely what he meant by "correctly"; he expected his students to do everything just as he had taught them, and if they did not, he would remove the instruments from their hands and finish the operation himself. From Gross, Glenn learned the value of mastering procedural detail and of applying the same rigor to the simplest and most complex surgical cases.

Glenn and Donald enjoy a record snowfall in March 1969 in Boston, where the Geelhoeds moved for medical residencies at Harvard Medical School.

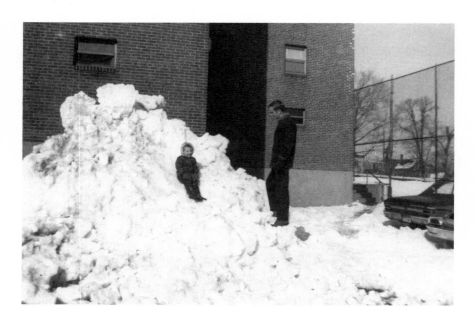

Glenn also saw in Gross a serious professional who knew how to have fun. Arriving for formal dinner one snowy evening at Gross's hilltop home in the Boston suburb of Framingham, Glenn asked who used the American Flyer sleds leaning against the porch—and suppressed laughter when Gross admitted that he did. (Because Gross had shared that secret, Glenn was the one he called some weeks later when he injured a wrist sledding and needed a cast put on it, no questions asked.)

Of all the storied physicians with whom Glenn studied at Harvard, none loomed larger than Franny Moore. When *Time* magazine published an article about trailblazing surgeons in a 1963 issue, its cover was a portrait of Moore under the legend, "If They Can Operate, You're Lucky." A residency tour under Moore wasn't just the all-absorbing study of surgery, Glenn would write later. It was also "a study of the chief and emulating his leadership in all personal and professional qualities."

Moore was exacting with his protégés and ambitious for his institution; he wanted both to be the best by every measure. He preferred that doctors on his team not be married, but if they were, he expected their spouses to put the doctors' careers first, whatever the spouses' own callings. Moore called Glenn "Dr. Geelhoed" but Sally "*Mrs.* Geelhoed." Only occasionally did the surgeon-in-chief reveal a softer side: When Glenn brought little Donald by the hospital, Moore would stop to joke with the boy and tousle his fair hair.

In most instances, Moore felt he knew better than his subordinates what was best for them. If they did not agree, he did not take it well. In 1970, in part thanks to Moore's influence, Glenn was offered a position at the National Cancer Institute of the federal National Institutes of Health in the Washington, D.C., suburbs. After working at NIH, Moore advised, Glenn should return to Harvard and punch his ticket through other prestigious postings—make a traditional ascent through institutional medicine, as Moore had done.

Glenn understood that being one of Moore's "fair-haired boys" might propel him far, but along a path that suited Moore more than it might suit him. Glenn had already glimpsed the possibilities of another path, a more winding, adventurous journey through disciplines beyond medicine, to exotic destinations where he felt profoundly needed and rewarded. In Moore's plan for him, Glenn saw what he called "slices of life." In his own plans and aspirations, he saw the whole globe.

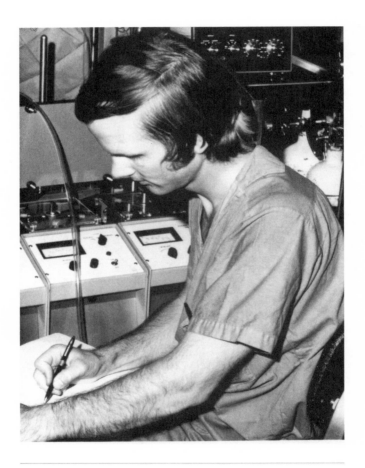

Glenn works on a research project during his fellowship at the federal National Institutes of Health, Bethesda, Maryland.

CHAPTER SIX

Around Barriers and Over Bridges

TO GLENN, THE ROCKVILLE, MARYLAND, TOWNHOUSE SEEMED BOTH
flimsy and overpriced. But it had much that he and Sally needed to ease the
move from Boston in spring 1970. Donald and Michael would have a bedroom to share and a next-door neighbor as their childcare provider. A short
commute to Bethesda took both Doctors Geelhoed to promising new jobs.
Glenn became a clinical associate in the surgery branch of the National Cancer Institute. Sally joined the Armed Forces Institute of Pathology, where she
worked with some of the top practitioners in military medicine.

Glenn remembers bright spots in the first months after the family's move:
stimulating work at NIH, sightseeing trips and hikes. But while the children
thrived and each parent prospered professionally, the couple struggled.

Decades later, Donald Geelhoed would describe Glenn and Sally as "two
headstrong medical students" who perhaps should never have wed. Donald
had barely entered elementary school and Michael still was in diapers when
the marriage broke apart.

Throughout Geelhoed family history as Glenn knew it, there never had
been a divorce, a separation, or even a really good fight. Marrying for life "was
how I was programmed," he once wrote. "It was how things were supposed
to go." In his life to that point, Glenn had attained what he desired through

a combination of intellect, hard work and sheer will. But in the summer of 1971, it became bitterly clear that he could not make some things—Sally, family, love—go as he wished they would.

Over the decades since, Glenn has consciously and probably unconsciously walled off memories of that time. What he always had imagined with Sally—two gifted physicians with soaring careers whose growing family would delight them—was disintegrating around him. He could hardly imagine then what he prefers not to remember now. The legal bones of it are somewhere in the attic: cartons of court papers, pleadings, decrees. He cannot bring himself to review the documents and only haltingly recalls what they describe.

Relatives sympathetic to Glenn fill in some of the details. Glenn's sisters tell how Sally took the boys "in the middle of the night" to her parents' home in Ohio; how Glenn pursued in a cross-country chase, left Ohio with Michael "wearing only his diaper," and drove to Michigan; how Glenn was arrested after bringing Michael to his parents, who drove the toddler back to Maryland while Glenn briefly was held in a Grand Rapids jail (where, true to his character, he passed a share of the night tending a cellmate's lacerated scalp).

The rest of the story, as nearly as it can be reconstructed, is a painful jumble of accusations—of duplicity, endangerment, faithlessness—hurled by onetime partners who had become combatants. Glenn sees the struggle as an extended assault. He becomes agitated and vocal when it is described as "she said, he said," as if he shares equally in the guilt and blame. What's clear to those close to the unhappiness is that Glenn has suffered it more than resolved it.

Donald remained with his mother in Ohio. Glenn returned to Maryland with Michael. It would be years before the brothers saw each other again, and before either boy saw the parent with whom he did not live. After rounds of legal wrangling, the divorce granted in 1974 brought an end more than a resolution. It had taken a toll on everyone: Sally, Donald, Michael and Glenn.

By then, Glenn had fashioned another family setting, one that accommodated the long hours and frequent travels of his medical career. He and Michael moved in with Dave and Mary VanderHart, fellow Calvin College graduates who attended the same Washington, D.C., church the Geelhoeds did and who helped care for Michael along with Laura, their daughter of the

same age. (A few years later the families would put down deeper roots, moving together into a comfortable brick house on a wooded, creek-laced property in Derwood, Maryland.)

In Franny Moore's estimation, his protégé had spent enough time gaining Washington-area experience and should return to the career path Moore envisioned at Harvard and the Brigham. Glenn remembers his nervousness when breaking the news to Moore that, because he had a good family setting for Michael as well as rewarding work in the Washington area, he would not be coming back to Boston.

The divorce, and the way it came about, had staggered Glenn's confidence that he could pursue any promising career and still be an adequate father. That the marriage had failed was as unchangeable as it was undeniable. But he still was a father; he still had Michael (and hope for having Donald as well). He was not willing to jeopardize what was left of his family to make the move back to Boston.

Moore made it clear he thought Glenn foolish to put "what might be best for children" above what certainly would be best for a promising surgeon. It took no imagination for Glenn to know he had fallen in Moore's regard.

He also believed he had made the right choice.

⸻ ⸝⸝⸝ ⸻

On September 12, 1977, Alice Geelhoed canned peaches, labeling batches to give to each of her children and keeping only a few for her own use. On September 13, she suffered a heart attack. Her children remember her joking gently, "I never even knew I had a heart" until the excruciating pain of its failure. She lingered for thirty hours after the attack, enough time for all four children to get to her bedside.

After Alice's death, Glenn says, relatives discovered a row of Mason jars she kept on shelves underneath the stairs at the family home. The jars contained coins and a few one- and five-dollar bills and were marked with names: Milly, Shirley . . . It was the money Alice had saved from her household budget and socked away, for others who might need it.

Like Glenn Geelhoed, Dr. Paul Shorb was a gifted surgeon with a blue-chip medical education. Shorb had been at George Washington University for a decade when he heard that "a star" was coming to the university from the NIH. Shorb remembers thinking skeptically, *I've heard that before.* But when he met Glenn, Shorb says, "I was absolutely blown away by the guy's brilliance," by his depth and breadth of knowledge and his obvious gifts as a teacher and a speaker. In 1977, Shorb was on the three-man medical faculty panel that voted to recommend Glenn for tenure.

With the divorce behind him and with Derwood as his life's anchor, Glenn threw himself into work, pursuing an ambitious schedule of teaching and operating at GWU while managing frequent domestic and international trips for lectures and visiting professorships. During a two-month stretch of 1977, he made two circumnavigations of the globe, one through Africa, India and the Far East and one through Southeast Asia. In one of the year-end letters he sends annually to relatives and friends, he described a typical re-entry after travels: "Within a few hours of arrival in Washington, I was back to operating, lecturing and carrying on the academic surgical career that seems to run a brisk pace all its own—with or without me."

Others at GWU took a different view. Increasingly, physicians and staff complained to administrators that they could not find Glenn when he was supposed to be on call, when needed for a consult or for postoperative care of his patients. Recalling those years, Glenn avoids the words "professional jealousy" and "academic competition," but the ideas float just under the surface.

Dr. Joseph Giordano (a GWU surgery resident with Glenn and later head of GWU's surgery department) recalls being "on the receiving end" of Glenn's transitions from GWU to his next trip. "Glenn would call me as he was going out the door: 'Joe, take care of this, and I'll be back in a week.' One particular time, he had six transplant patients in the house, and then he left. Things went well, but I was not really a transplant surgeon, so it was a little difficult to follow his patients. In retrospect, it seems clear that Glenn's niche was international medicine. He really didn't have the desire for day-to-day

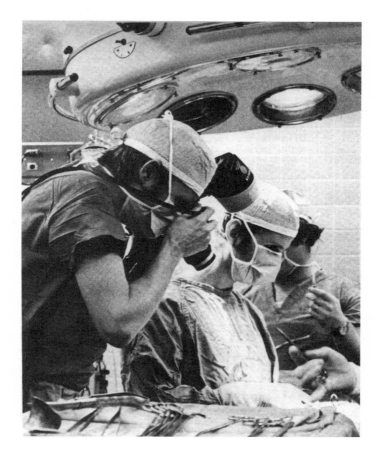

At George Washington University Medical Center, a photographer documents a 1974 kidney transplant operation performed by Glenn and a team of colleagues.

care of patients. For him, there was a certain boredom; it didn't excite him."

When some patient complaints turned into malpractice charges, Glenn was eager to fight them. He was convinced the claims were baseless; GWU officials were not so sure. Over time, the hospital quietly settled a number of suits, at a cost to its self-insured malpractice fund that hospital officials put at hundreds of thousands of dollars.

If Glenn's work sometimes drew fire from associates and administrators, it was simultaneously drawing accolades from the scientific and medical communities. For 1986, he was named a traveling scholar of the James IV

Association of Surgeons, a society that promotes international exchanges and collaborations among surgeons. The honor came with a stipend that allowed Glenn to spend most of two months traveling, teaching and studying. Over the course of the scholar experience, Glenn gave lectures, trained physicians and residents, assisted in operations and ward rounds, and explored cultures in four very different environments: South Africa, Sweden, Pakistan and the United Kingdom.

For the "surgeon-internationalist" that Glenn was becoming, the experience was a feast. In Sweden he consulted with eminent physicians and scientists, some of whom worked at the Nobel Institute. In Britain, he studied the National Health Service, compared it to the U.S. approach to health care, and concluded that both too often elevated bureaucracy over patient care. In Pakistan, he lectured at the plush, new Aga Khan University Medical College, then toured the Karachi slums, where health care ranged from haphazard to nonexistent and where the infant mortality rate topped 10 percent.

In South Africa, Glenn stepped into the passion play of the waning years of apartheid. He met with prominent figures who were publicly challenging the system: Archbishop Desmond Tutu, political reformer the Reverend Dr. Allan Boesak. But just as powerful were the private meetings with ambitious medical students at the University of Capetown's Groote Schuur Hospital. They vented their fury at being barred from choice medical posts because they were "colored," Indian or mixed-race.

Writing about the South Africa trip, Glenn emphasized that he had neither claimed expertise nor formed opinions on the politics of "this beautiful and troubled land." But he decried the "dreary dominion of skin color" that kept so many citizens from reaching their full potential.

Glenn's final report on the James IV experience ran more than 220 pages, counting text, itineraries and appendices. Its last lines left no doubt that, while medicine would always be his profession, he believed international medicine was an even higher calling. Being a James IV Scholar, Glenn wrote, enabled him to "go around barriers and over bridges. There are any number of the former and precious few of the latter among the peoples of this small planet. Some of those barriers could be breached if there were bridges enough.

Disease, hunger and want isolate people naturally, and political, economic and religious systems may also do so . . . But the healing art is a nearly ideal, transportable skill across all artificial barriers among humans."

A nearly ideal, transportable skill. If Glenn needed further proof of his convictions about the healing arts, he found it in fall 1987 in an African village just big enough to have a name: Assa.

Across central Africa, where huge swaths of land have changed hands and names repeatedly over centuries, countries Glenn once visited are no longer on the map. One great, roadless tract covers parts of the Central African Republic, southern Sudan and the Democratic Republic of Congo (formerly known as Zaire and, before that, Belgian Congo). Yet for all the shifting boundaries that subdivide it, the region still is known by its traditional name, Zandeland, ancestral home of the Azande tribe.

Within Zandeland lies the world's second largest rain forest, the Ituri Forest, a 63,000-square-kilometer marvel that captured Glenn's imagination as he flew over it. "It keeps on going forever," he wrote in a journal. "With just a different tint, it is the ocean, spread out on all sides on a flat earth as far as the eye can see to each horizon. It is endless broccoli."

To the east of the Ituri Forest is the village of Nyankunde, home to the Centre Medical Evangelique (CME). A missionary hospital sponsored by European religious groups, the CME is the chief source of medical services and training for an area the size of France, with a population topping eight million. To the west and north of the Ituri, more than six hundred miles from Nyankunde by air, is the bush outpost called Assa.

Since the 1930s, small bands of U.S. missionaries had been coming to Assa to live, build and teach. 1980 marked the arrival of the Downing family: Diane, a nurse; her husband, David, a builder and surgical technician; son Scott and daughters Dawn and Shelly. The village was little more than a school building, a church and an air strip, which were ringed by clusters of family huts. Everywhere, Diane witnessed the desperate need for health care

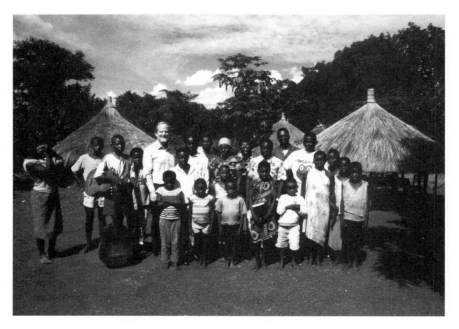

Glenn poses with villagers during a medical mission to Assa, Congo.

and high rates of tuberculosis, leprosy, malaria and malnutrition. But most striking was the incidence of hypothyroidism.

In patients with hypothyroidism, the lobes of the thyroid gland—a butterfly-shaped endocrine gland that straddles the airway in the neck—enlarge to try to trap iodine that the body lacks. The enlargement results in growths called goiters. Milder cases can be treated with iodine-bearing oral medications; more severe cases require surgical removal of the gland.

The villagers of Assa suffered hypothyroidism at its most extreme, for a perfect storm of reasons. The volcanic soil in which they grew subsistence crops held almost no iodine. The chief food crop they grew, cassava root, contained non-lethal amounts of cyanide, a chemical that actually blocked the body's use of iodine, compounding the problem. Villagers' usual evening meal was pounded cassava root—a filling, high-fiber but low-nutrition mush that they flavored with peanut butter, hot peppers and palm oil. Consequently, nearly all of the people of Assa suffered from malnutrition, and as a whole, the population had one of the world's highest rates of hypothyroidism.

Throughout Assa and surrounding villages, the Downings saw hypo-thyroidism's effects. Adults were lethargic and weak, their metabolisms so depressed that daily life and work were exhausting. Diane estimated that 95 percent of the population had goiters, many so large and disfiguring that they impeded breathing. Women suffered reduced fertility and struggled to bear the healthy children who afforded both status and household help.

In children, the effects were even more cruel. Hypothyroidism retarded both mental and physical development, causing a condition known as cre-tinism. From birth or very young ages, many of Assa's children exhibited worsening signs of cretinism: stunted growth, reduced mental capacity, muteness. Into adulthood, many never matured sexually, and some never lost their baby teeth. If females with cretinism did become pregnant, many bore cretin babies, or they died because their stunted bodies could not accommodate childbirth.

With villagers serving as construction crews, the Downings built Assa a basic medical center, with an operating room, delivery room, patient ward, clinic and pharmacy. They encouraged visits from medical mission teams, especially surgeons who could help the most desperate goiter patients. Dur-ing a visit back to the United States, Diane sought out Dr. Timothy Harri-son, a renowned endocrine researcher and thyroid surgeon, and explained Assa's plight.

In 1984, Harrison came to Assa and helped the Downings launch the Goiter Project, a treatment and study initiative to see if injecting villagers with long-acting iodine would reduce or eliminate their thyroid disease. The project began with 423 patients. Diane recorded each one's symptoms, wrap-ping their throats in tissue paper and tracing the outlines of goiters. Then each received a simple, inexpensive injection of iodine mixed with poppy seed oil, which the body slowly would absorb over the course of three to five years.

Within months after the first injections, blood tests showed thyroid hor-mones returning to healthy levels, and measurements showed goiters were shrinking. As Diane evaluated every study participant every six months, the good news became even better. Villagers were recovering energy and fertility;

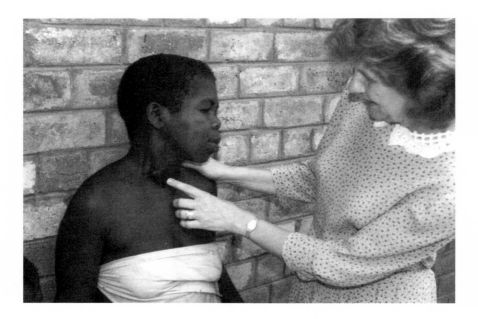

Nurse Diane Downing examines Umbatiole, a resident of Assa, Congo, after an operation that removed her thyroid gland. When Downing and her family came to Assa as missionaries, Diane estimated that 95 percent of the population had goiters, a growth that occurs when the thyroid gland enlarges to try to trap iodine that the body lacks.

some cretins who had been mute and largely helpless were learning to speak and do simple tasks. When several women who had received the iodine gave birth and not one bore a cretin, the study protocol was changed to provide injections to all women of childbearing age who came in for prenatal care.

The Downings and Harrison were ecstatic at the success and eager to expand the project. Harrison made plans to return to Assa in 1987 and told the Downings he'd bring along another endocrine-surgery expert, a onetime student of Harrison's at the University of Michigan Medical School, a doctor named Glenn Geelhoed.

For two weeks, Glenn operated on patients with large, hard-to-excise goiters, while also helping to expand the Goiter Project in Assa and surrounding villages. The experience was "scientifically stimulating and medically very rewarding," Glenn wrote in his journal. Though the time passed too quickly, the experience rekindled the fire he had first felt for this kind of work, two decades earlier in Nigeria. "These were very needy and neglected people and had very few means of fending for themselves," Glenn wrote. He would return to Assa, he told the Downings, as soon and as often as he could.

By the mid-1980s, Paul Shorb was a respected veteran among GWU surgeons. He was also a recovering alcoholic who talked candidly about completing rehab in 1981, after years of colleagues "looking the other way" and covering his cases instead of urging him to face his problems.

The fight with his own demons left Shorb fascinated by the question of "what leads able people into self-destructive patterns." In late 1989, when GWU administrators convened a faculty committee to review Glenn's performance, Shorb agreed to accompany Glenn to committee proceedings and assist with his defense. Giordano, then Glenn's colleague and later head of GWU's surgery department, says the committee was formed because administrators believed "Glenn had to change his ways to continue to function as a practicing surgeon." While the committee investigated, Glenn was not permitted to operate.

Shorb (who retired from GWU in 2001) still remembers the review process in detail: months of weekly two- to three-hour meetings in conference rooms as the committee pored over cases, reviewing documents and taking testimony recorded by a transcriptionist. As one of GWU's ranking specialists in endocrine surgery, Glenn had done countless successful thyroidectomies. Because the operation involves making an incision in the neck at the throat to remove the thyroid gland, it carries the risk of interfering with the recurrent laryngeal nerve, potentially causing difficulties in voice use and timber, coughing and breathing. Cases before the committee included two of Glenn's thyroid operation patients who had received settlements from GWU for recurrent laryngeal nerve injury.

Another case before the committee concerned a patient who, because he had hemophilia, was given a blood clotting medication in preparation for an emergency hernia operation. Rather than scheduling a later operation to remove the patient's thyroid tumor, Glenn removed it after the hernia operation, under cover of the same clotting medication. Glenn then left on a previously scheduled international trip. Despite transfusions, the patient did not recover and died in the intensive care unit. Shorb says other physicians on the case strongly disagreed with Glenn's call and resented inheriting the management of this patient. At the time and to this day, Glenn believes he was right to do the thyroid operation.

In February 1990, the committee produced its recommendation: that Dr. Geelhoed be allowed to resume his surgical career if he agreed to certain restrictions about asking other physicians to cover his patients and leaving town after performing operations. As Shorb recalls it, the GWU hospital medical director thanked the committee for its hard work and considered its conclusions "for about five minutes" before declaring that Glenn would have to apply to regain surgical privileges and that he would recommend against their restoration.

To Glenn, the ruling was unfathomable, a miscarriage of justice and a repudiation of all he had accomplished at GWU. Shorb says he understood the administration's choice, but still felt that "Glenn had been badly wronged by this process. Why go through a charade if you knew what the result was going to be?" Shorb encouraged Glenn to appeal the ruling to a higher body at the university.

Within days after the ruling, Glenn was flying over the Ituri Forest, on a long-arranged trip to the Congo that now felt especially like a homecoming. "Dave and Diane Downing and all my other good friends welcomed my return to the wonderful environment of Assa," he wrote in his journal. "I walked in the dry-season forest, awakened to the cacophony of the bird song at dawn, and settled into the medical work and investigation of the Goiter Project."

On frequent treks into the bush, Glenn's Congolese hosts taught him centuries-old tricks of tracking. Between the locals' spears and Glenn's rifle, they brought back enough guinea fowl, waterbuck and Cape buffalo to feed the whole village for weeks. The outings "brought me even closer to my friends who share this instinct of the hunter-gatherer with me," Glenn wrote in his journal. "I also have a greater appreciation of their adaptation to circumstances in which life is hard but still to be enjoyed."

A week before what would have been his appeal date at GWU, Glenn told Shorb he would not pursue it. Instead he was going on sabbatical to London to earn a degree in tropical medicine. At that moment, GWU, his institutional home for nearly two decades, seemed all about confines, limits on what he could do. In Africa, he had seen the limitlessness of a doctor's place in the developing world: unending work, boundless need, perpetual learning, maximum freedom.

In retrospect, Giordano feels that as a GWU staff surgeon in the 1970s and 1980s, "Glenn had not found his niche. What he really wanted to do was be a world traveler and educator and do international work. And once he found that, he has done it in spades."

Late 1990 found Glenn back at GWU with an office, a salary and his tenured professor of surgery title; he never sought to reclaim surgical privileges there. With the additional title of professor of international medical education, he would operate essentially as a one-man clearinghouse for international medical missions. Constrained from teaching surgery in GWU's operating rooms, he found other ORs—the more remote and threadbare, the better—where he could teach local practitioners as well as medical students and colleagues traveling with him.

Glenn's 1990 year-end letter describes the life change simply: "Turning away from the injustices of GWU's interference with my academic surgical career, to resume it later elsewhere."

He could dwell on the events that brought him to that crossroads, the barriers. Or he could fashion a new life map, building bridges to wherever he wished.

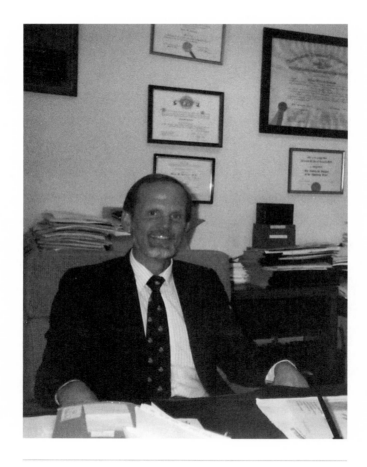

Professor of Surgery and Professor of International Medical Education: Glenn in 1991 in his George Washington University office.

CHAPTER SEVEN

Riding More than One Horse

GLENN HAD HEARD THE TALE BEFORE AND WOULD REPEAT IT FOR years after. But at the time of the upheaval at GWU, he found special meaning in a story about Benvenuto Cellini.

In sixteenth-century Italy, Cellini was known as a brilliant sculptor, a Renaissance man, and a connoisseur of life's pleasures. He was not yet thirty when he contracted syphilis. As the disease advanced and Cellini weakened, an unscrupulous associate named Sbietta talked Cellini into a land deal that would benefit Sbietta at Cellini's death. Eager to have his payday, Sbietta and his wife invited Cellini to a dinner that Cellini described in his autobiography:

"Sbietta's wife had set before me plates, and porringers, and saucers different from the others," he wrote. "The sauce was very well made and pleasant to the taste ... I could not imagine why she urged me so persistently to eat." Heading home after the meal, "I had not gone three miles before I felt as though my stomach was on fire." Cellini's conclusion: "They must have administered a dose of sublimate in the sauce"—sublimate, also known as mercury.

The poison caused severe intestinal inflammation and bleeding and put Cellini in bed for months. While the mercury-laced sauce was not enough to kill him, it was just enough to cure his syphilis. He lived to the ripe old age of seventy-one.

When one of Cellini's royal patrons heard the story, he offered to punish the would-be assassins. Cellini wouldn't hear of it and explained his choice with this proverb: "God send us evil that may work us good."

⸎

Within two years after the ruling on Glenn's surgical privileges, the officials he held most responsible all had left GWU. Glenn never believed the officials were justified in ending his academic surgical career there. After they did, he saw his options clearly: "You can curse God and die, and that would be a fairly swift and easy end to your miseries. It's a long, hard trek the other way, to try to re-create something good of that which is a given." At first, he wondered if his new career course was just a default position—what his Midwestern forebears would have called "making a silk purse out of a sow's ear." But over time, it felt more and more like what he'd been destined to do all along.

Since early in his GWU career, Glenn had lent his voice to causes that engaged him. For the organization International Physicians for the Prevention of Nuclear War (IPPNW), he addressed a symposium on the consequences of a nuclear attack on Washington, D.C., sharing the dais with high-profile physicians and scientists including vaccine pioneer Dr. Jonas Salk and physicist Carl Sagan. A *Washington Post* article captured the scene: "With a spotlight sinking his eyes in deep shadows, molding his cheekbones and shadowing his long beard, Dr. Glenn Geelhoed looked as well as sounded like a prophet of doom yesterday as he told 1,000 physicians that any hopes they may have of healing victims of a nuclear attack on Washington are meaningless." To silence from the shocked crowd, Glenn noted that given the hospital's location between the Pentagon and the White House, "In the event of a thermonuclear strike, we will be part of a crater eighty meters deep." For its efforts, the IPPNW was awarded a Nobel Peace Prize.

In the hours no longer spent teaching and operating at GWU, Glenn explored other ways to fulfill the childhood catechism that said he was "saved to serve." He joined in activities of two other organizations that also earned Nobel Peace Prizes: Medecins Sans Frontiers (Doctors

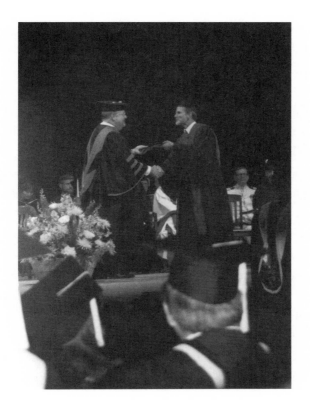

Glenn receives the first of several advanced degrees he would complete while on the GWU faculty: a master's degree in international affairs from GWU's Elliott School of International Affairs.

Without Borders) and the International Campaign to Ban Landmines. And the professor again became the student, pursuing advanced degrees in fields he felt would help him serve the globe's patients. During the first year after his GWU status changed, he completed a master's degree in international relations and started a master's degree in epidemiology.

Early in 1991, Glenn traveled to Paris to receive a singular honor: induction into France's venerable Academie de Chirurgie. In a wry notation in his journal, Glenn wrote that he wasn't entirely sure membership was an honor, "because the original members all lost their heads." The surgical society, the oldest in France, was founded in 1731 by King Louis XV's personal surgeon, then dissolved in 1793 when the French Revolution cost many bourgeoisie doctors their status (and some their lives).

Joking aside, Geelhoed embraced the chance to be an *associé etranger* (foreign associate) of the academy. Induction, in a grand ceremony in an ornate palace, provided a well-timed affirmation of his standing in the profession as well as a chance to connect with counterparts from around the world. The visit to France reunited Glenn with Dr. Charles Proye, a storied endocrine surgeon who had nominated Glenn for the academy honor.

Proye was the very definition of a bon vivant: a rugby-playing, Kronenbourg-chugging activist known throughout Europe as a brilliant surgeon. He appreciated colleagues with whom he could share the exquisite ironies of life and the cellar selections he modestly billed as "ordinary peasant wines." Glenn and the equally adventurous Proye had frequently run into each other at international surgeons' conclaves, where they would slip away from work sessions to scuba dive or stay up late sharing philosophical conversations. After the academy ceremony, the two took the high-speed TGV train from Paris to Lille, the Proye family's hometown.

For the six weeks he spent in Lille, Glenn stepped into the rarified world his French counterparts inhabited. Proye and his colleagues practiced at the leading edge of their surgical specialty; they were, Glenn knew, the western world's ideal of success in their field. Beyond the hospital, the surgeons' lives were equally privileged: Many evenings they went from the operating suite to an elegant soiree or sumptuous meal, as Proye's family ran L'Huitriere, a Michelin-starred Lille restaurant.

Proye dropped broad hints to his American guest: "One could do worse, *mon ami*, than to join us here in Lille." But when Glenn accepted the invitation to operate with Proye, the differences in their approaches were striking. As he later recalled it, "I'm working with Proye. I'm proceeding swiftly and directly to isolate and occlude the central adrenal vein in a patient with a potentially deadly adrenal tumor. And he says to those assisting us, 'Look, it's so American. He goes right to where the problem is!' And I am thinking, 'Well, what else is there?' But for him, there was such emphasis on the exercise of the technique, the performance and display of the anatomic dissection. It may have made no contribution to the patient's welfare; it had more hazardous than therapeutic effect. There was less concern about the outcome than about, 'Voila! Look at what I have just done!'"

Glenn saw the charms of the life Proye led: professional stature, creature comforts, traveling first-class. But he couldn't picture himself long-term in such a "gold-headed-cane" environment. He also saw Proye and colleagues working on the same procedures and maladies repeatedly, and to him that felt less like perfecting an art than settling into a rut. Working in just one area of medicine, he told colleagues, was a sure prescription for obsolescence. He was more inclined toward what he called "riding more than one horse"— practicing across a number of disciplines, advancing and synthesizing them for a multiplier effect.

Since high school, he had chafed at the notion that focusing on one area of knowledge meant not pursuing others. Now he rejected the idea completely with a phrase he delighted in repeating: "I refuse to live my life according to the limits of another's imagination."

To explain what he meant, he recalled a scene from *Pretty Woman*, the movie about the improbable romance between a business magnate and a streetwalker. "Remember when Richard Gere comes up to Julia Roberts and asks, 'What's your name?' And she responds, 'What do you want it to be?' It's like that with me. Someone asks, 'What are you? Are you a transplant surgeon?' 'Yes, if you need a transplant surgeon.' 'Are you an endocrine surgeon?' 'Yeah, honey, that too.' 'A cancer surgeon?' 'Yes.' But if someone demands of me, 'Well, which is it? Decide!' my response is, 'I choose not to choose.'"

Glenn continued to travel the United States and the world as a lecturer and visiting professor. The more time he spent at premier medical institutions with paying clientele, the greater his conviction that this was not where he was most needed. But the speaking engagements proved useful in advancing his greater interest: When he invited audience members to join him on medical missions, he almost always found a few takers; and the speaker fees helped him pay for mission supplies and airfares.

Summer 1993 found both of Glenn's sons grown and through college. Donald was working in law enforcement in Florida; Michael had married and moved to Texas with his new bride, Judy. With an empty nest at Derwood and no fixed schedule at GWU, Glenn traveled at will.

He answered the call when global relief organizations sought doctors to go to the sites of natural disasters. He joined in mission trips organized by medical organizations or religious groups, but their approaches often struck him as overly bureaucratic or paternalistic. So whenever possible, he organized his own mission trips to his own specifications, handling everything from recruiting participants and scrounging supplies to obtaining visas and booking air charters. His idea of a prime mission location was anywhere other groups deemed too remote or dangerous to visit, where he and his team could train local medical personnel while treating the world's poorest patients.

At the GWU medical school, Glenn's office was moved from the surgical floor to an administrative wing. When students came looking for the Center for International Medical Education, they found one small office overflowing with papers, and one wiry professor brimming with enthusiasm.

John Sutter, a former firefighter and social worker, chose GWU for medical school because he was interested in international work. But when he researched one of the school's formal study-abroad programs, Sutter says, "It was basically people staying in high-end hotels in wealthy Middle Eastern countries. It didn't really sound like what I wanted.

"Then another medical student told me, 'There's a guy named Geelhoed that you need to talk to.' I found his office, knocked and got no answer. I probably did that every day for three weeks—never an answer. Finally I go there, the door's ajar, I knock, and he calls out, 'Come on in!' There's basically just his desk and boxes everywhere, things all over the place. We talked, and it became clear he had been out of the country as I was trying to find him.

"I told him I knew a little Spanish and wanted to do medical mission work in Central and South America. I'm going on with my spiel, and he interrupts me and says, 'See that picture? It's K2 in the Himalayas,'" the second highest mountain on earth. "And he's like, 'Why don't you go there with me next summer?' It was the complete opposite of what I was thinking about doing." It was also the first of several medical mission trips Sutter would take with Glenn.

Over the many years and miles, Glenn has developed certain routines for the trips and certain expectations for participants. He books the flight itineraries, lodging and in-country arrangements and divides the cost among team members (though during the mission he often treats them to a special meal or tour, as his guests). He tells team members he will never donate the first dollar of their trip costs. But if participants raise all they can and still come up short, he sometimes helps cover the difference. At speaking events, during audience Q-and-A sessions, when he is asked what entity underwrites his missions, he often says, "my American Express card." Though he is grateful when admirers of his work send donations, medicines and supplies for missions, he refuses to do fundraising.

Glenn advises team members that the two checked bags each traveler is allowed must be filled with medical supplies, so all of their personal effects must fit into their carry-on luggage. At Derwood, on the eve of each trip, he provides pizza and beer at a packing and unpacking party, during which he coaches participants on how to load and weigh the bright blue duffels of supplies, and coaxes them to leave behind such personal "essentials" as blow-dryers.

Organizations that sponsor medical-mission programs typically have fixed requirements about a participant's age, education and expertise. Many specifically bar medical students from performing certain tasks or traveling to locations deemed hazardous. By contrast, Glenn's process for assembling medical teams relies more on intuition than regimentation. On past missions, he has taken team members as young as sixteen and doctors retired from medical practice, some people with decades of health-care experience and others with none.

While Glenn selects team members partly on the basis of what they have done previously, he is at least as interested in what they are willing to do— whether they're willing, as he says, "to jump into the deep end of the pool" and tackle any challenge that arises. Though some bridle at the term, Glenn intends no insult when he calls mission candidates "wannabes." He does, however, divide them into two camps. He's wary of those who want to be on trips for what he considers the wrong reasons: to act out a savior complex, score a great adventure, or break from a life that's lacking. He's looking for recruits who want to be on the trips for the same reasons he does: to serve and learn.

Glenn warns would-be participants that the developing world will test their flexibility in fluid situations and their capacity to manage frustration. He commends them for wanting to go, serve, make a difference. He cautions that when they see the enormity of the need, they may feel despair. Above all, before they go, he insists that participants unpack one more piece of baggage: any sense that they are superior to, or separate from, the people they will meet. At more departures than he can count, he has offered essentially the same thoughts:

> *These people we will meet are not at all like us; they are us. They are friends and neighbors you have not yet met. They may look different in terms of trivia such as skin color or language, geographic boundaries or economic situations. They may seem so different that you don't know how to relate to them. But look at the most fundamental things you have that you'd want to give up last: your children, your health, your hope. In this, we all are the same.*
>
> *When you were young, your mother told you, 'Eat your peas; there are children in the world starving.' If you were a smart aleck, maybe you challenged her: 'Starving children? Name three.' Well, that is my job, to introduce you to the three, so you are in some very direct way responsible for them, your brothers and sisters.*
>
> *When you meet them, one of the things you will find out quickly is that these people have resources — not like coffee or gold or oil that's been taken away from them, but resiliency and resourcefulness. And that is how they can become instructors to us. What we teach and give to them will pale in comparison to what we learn and receive from them — what I call gifts from the poor.*

Gifts from the poor. Glenn cannot remember when he first used that phrase to name what he derives from missions in the developing world. Some are gifts of character: how to thrive despite deprivation, to summon strength in the face of suffering. Some are gifts of experience: friendships with inspiring figures, memorable patients and selfless healers. Some are gifts of enlightenment: learning to appreciate the beauty and wisdom of other cultures but also to stand against cultural practices that dehumanize and destroy. From every medical mission, Glenn, his colleagues and his students return laden with stories of these humbling, disturbing, life-changing gifts.

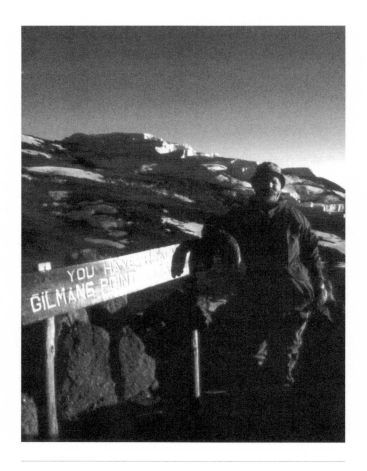

During his Fulbright Scholar travels in 1996, Glenn reached "the roof of Africa": the summit of Mount Kilimanjaro in Tanzania.

Chapter Eight

The Year of Fulbrightness

A SON OF MIDDLE AMERICA, TRANSFORMED BY TIME SPENT ABROAD—
before that was Glenn Geelhoed's story, it was Bill Fulbright's.

As a graduate student at Oxford University, J. William Fulbright developed a passion for international affairs. He returned to the United States, studied and taught law, then ran for Congress from his native Arkansas. During more than three decades on Capitol Hill, Fulbright profoundly influenced America's foreign policy. In 1946, Senator Fulbright introduced legislation creating an international educational exchange program for scholars. Since then, the program that bears his name has operated in 155 countries and supported nearly 300,000 Fulbrighters, including, in 1996, Glenn Geelhoed.

Glenn used the Fulbright stipend to do more of what he'd been doing already: medical research and service, studying and teaching, with some running and adventuring thrown in. By the end of what he breezily dubbed "my Year of Fulbrightness," Glenn had logged travels through eight African nations and five Middle Eastern ones, plus a quick stop in Sri Lanka, a climb to the top of Tanzania's Mount Kilimanjaro, and a respectable finish in the 100th running of the Boston Marathon.

The experiences of that single year, like none before it, profoundly influenced Glenn's approach to international medicine. After 1996, he was headed down a different path. He was not content to take occasional medical missions organized by others; he was determined to lead frequent missions when and where he chose, and to make that the centerpiece of his life.

At every stop in the scholarship year, the Fulbright entree gave Glenn choice opportunities: deep-sea fishing charters and wildlife safaris, fine-wine suppers and Zambezi River rafting. But it also gave him a sharper view of the divide between the temporary-resident class—aid agencies, non-governmental organizations (NGOs), even visiting doctor/scholars—and the permanently destitute masses whose plight visitors came to address. While many of the people Glenn saw were living in poverty, a small, successful strata seemed to be living *off* poverty, or at least off of institutions built to assuage it.

Through a quarter-century in Washington, D.C., Glenn had seen plenty of social programs that were created to address a serious problem but over time became less about problem solving and more about self-preservation. In his Fulbright tour through developing nations, he saw this dynamic again. Relief and development agencies, religious and secular, had arrived with good intentions and generous aid grants. Their plans were stalled or compromised by corrupt and broken governments. Their money was not enough to seriously impact social ills—but still enough to hook locals on the notion of aid as entitlement and foreigners as charity dispensers.

The dilemma crystallized for Glenn in the nation the World Bank ranked as the world's poorest, Mozambique. Two questions seemed most pressing, Glenn wrote at the time: "How to go about helping this population in view of the numbing need and resources limited in supply and effectiveness, nearly all from foreign donation." And, compared to others who had come before, "How am I supposed to be different?"

If Glenn's Fulbright experience yielded a "gift from the poor," it was a refined sense of how *not* to serve them. Glenn still believed he should provide free medical care, but only in conjunction with training locals, so communities would eventually become less dependent on imported healers. He would work as he worked best, as a sole proprietor—no overhead, no oversight, ultimate control. Though he might still go on medical missions run by institutions, he vowed never to become one. The ultimate goal of his mission teams would be to work themselves out of a job.

In essays, letters and journals, Glenn recorded the memorable year. From the many volumes, three episodes in Mozambique stand out: A hit-and-run, a mugging, and a wild ride to a hospital along flood-ravaged train tracks.

On descent into Maputo, Mozambique, the jetliner circled the city three times, affording Glenn a good view of the former Portuguese colonial capital. "Though it may not be politically correct to speak of parts of the world as underdeveloped, there hardly seems a point in denying this special position of Mozambique," he wrote in his journal. "Post-colonial neglect, insufficient infrastructure, destabilizing capitalist neighbors, enervating aid from Western and Eastern blocs in turn, and, most particularly, brutal civil war for most of the two decades since independence resulted in a failed socialist state. Whatever the layering of reasons or blame for the nation's current predicament, it has become a laboratory for what can be done to turn the 'down and out' into the 'up and forward.'"

U.S. embassy personnel greeted Glenn at the airport and then settled him into the government car that would deliver him to his apartment for the Fulbright stay. Glenn described the scene in an essay:

We pulled out of the airport and into traffic following numerous vehicles whose license plates identified them as belonging to NGOs working in Mozambique, one of the leading aid recipients of the world, for cause. The streets were crowded with pedestrians attempting to run across traffic to the curbside markets lining the roads. We had hardly got under way when I saw a barefoot man wearing only shorts pushing a cart loaded with crated, empty

Coke bottles. An NGO car ahead of us was headed right for the cart and I braced myself for the noisy, spectacular crash that seemed inevitable.

As the driver of my car braked to a stop, things seemed to move in slow-motion. The NGO car's driver swerved to avoid hitting the cart—and in missing the cart, the car hit the man dead center with a sickening thud. The man was tossed into the air, cleared the roof of the car by more than a meter, then dropped flat out on the pavement with a loud crack and a bounce. The NGO car did not stop. For a moment the man lay motionless. I was about to get out and go to him when the man stirred and, in obvious pain, began crawling to the curb. "See, he is moving. He is going to be all right," said my car's driver as he pulled me back into the car, and the car back into traffic.

It occurred to me that the collision was not just physical but cultural—one of Mozambique's poorer citizens struck down by a vehicle from an agency here to aid the poor. No bottles were broken, although almost certainly bones were. In terms of supply, one seemed to have higher value than the other.

In the Fulbright scholar's apartment, running water was available for thirty minutes once a day, and it had to be boiled before use (on the stove's one working burner). When the power was not blinking off, it was surging, melting Glenn's electrical current adaptors. Glenn could comfortably forego for a few weeks the amenities that most Mozambicans went without constantly. But he could not give up one staple of his U.S. existence: his regular runs.

Figuring he'd combine exercise, errands and sightseeing, Glenn dressed in running shorts, shoes and a T-shirt lettered with a large "GEORGE WASH-INGTON." In a plastic grocery bag he could carry on his arm, he packed travel essentials: a Dictaphone for capturing sound, a Nikon camera plus film and batteries, traveler's checks, apartment keys, a notepad full of contacts and journal jottings. He would run along the picturesque seaside road to the bustling fish market. But first he should go to the money exchange, via a tree-lined road through a park.

It all happened so fast. Dropping from the tree in front of me was a man approximately twenty-five years old and dressed in a bright green T-shirt, trousers and what I noted to be relatively new running shoes two sizes too big. The focus of my attention, though, was the two-foot blade in his right hand. With the blade in stabbing position, he lunged at me. As I swerved to avoid the blade, a second man, armed with a bayonet, jumped from the bush behind me. He lunged from the rear as the first man grappled for the plastic bag wound around my left wrist.

Another slow-motion moment, as the plastic bag came apart and all three of us watched the valuables spill from it. The first man grabbed the camera and Dictaphone and tossed them to the man behind me. Then he inserted his blade under my watchband and tried to saw at the tough plastic. I recall thinking at that point, "They are more scared than I am." But I also had clear visions of the ward full of trauma and assault victims in Hospital Central de Maputo.

While the second man was distracted with the camera and Dictaphone, I broke from the first man and sprinted toward the main street. Neither assailant followed. Though well away, I could hear the first man, enraged, screaming, "Money! Money! Money!"

I flagged down a European woman driving her son and daughter in a Mercedes, and explained that I had just been robbed. She shrugged and said, "It happens all the time, and you surely don't expect the police to do anything about it." Nonetheless, she dropped me at the chief gendarmerie in Maputo.

There, an inspector spent more than an hour and a half preparing a one-paragraph report in florid Portuguese legalese. No request was made for location, description of assailants, witnesses, or any things I would consider fundamental to police work. But the inspector did ask, with only a passing interest, what could be the ultimate question: "Why were you here in the first place?"

Glenn dutifully reported the incident to U.S. embassy officials, who immediately scheduled him for a briefing on travel precautions.

As soon as he could get a replacement notepad, Glenn wrote down every detail of the events. An avid collector of metaphors, he particularly relished this one: a blade-wielding African pauper demanding "Money! Money! Money!" from a First-Worlder wearing the name Washington.

In an essay, Glenn pondered the connection between the scavenger crossing the road and the scholar going for a run. "The first resulted in risk to life and limb; the second resulted in a loss of excess property. In both instances, given the circumstances, it was considered an acceptable risk of doing business," he wrote. "Each illustrated a clash of cultures and values at the intersection of the helpers and the aided ones. How can this relationship evolve? Probably not efficiently, nor even gracefully at times, but we are here to try! God help each of us, and save us from each other."

Glenn first visited Mozambique in 1993, just months into the peace accord that ended fifteen brutal years of civil war. He went at the invitation of one of the preeminent surgeons in the war-scarred country: Dr. Paulo Ivo Albasini Teixeira Garrido.

When Ivo was born, his homeland still was a Portuguese colony. An exceptional student, he was in school at Maputo in 1969 when a letter-bomb blast killed Eduardo Mondlane, the pro-independence leader considered his country's George Washington. By the time Mozambique won independence in 1975, young Doctor Ivo was working in Hospital Central de Maputo as one of the few remaining doctors in the nation after most who had come from Portugal as medical students had fled.

But the ruling socialist FRELIMO party soon came under attack by anti-communist RENAMO forces, and in 1977 the young nation erupted in civil war. Beyond the military casualties, hundreds of thousands of civilians fell in crossfire or from landmines both factions planted indiscriminately.

One of a handful of surgeons still in the country, Ivo struggled to stem the carnage. In the darkest of the war years, he barely could find food for his family and hardly left the hospital for weeks on end. A friend and counselor to Mozambican president Samora Machel, Ivo had met with Machel and shared hopeful talk about national unity just days before Machel perished in a suspicious plane crash, in October 1986.

Glenn knew well that a talented surgeon could work almost anywhere. He admired Ivo enormously for remaining in his shattered homeland. As soon as the Fulbright was his, Glenn laid plans to spend part of the scholar tour with Ivo, helping as he could with the healing of Mozambique.

For two weeks in Maputo, Glenn operated on patients and taught practitioners at the capital's central hospital. He coached faculty at the University Eduardo Mondlane medical school and advised government officials on restoring health systems. On Friday nights he dined with Ivo's extended family, enjoying Ivo's mother's home cooking and his father's Frank Sinatra recordings. When the nation's minister of health asked Glenn and Ivo to assess health needs in the countryside, the two doctors set out to cover hundreds of miles from Maputo in the south to the far-north Niassa province.

Three years into postwar reconstruction, Mozambique had a shaky national airline that flew to some cities only once weekly; many bridges still were bombed-out or half-repaired, and many roads still rubble. Despite and around the obstacles, Ivo guided Glenn through his country. They visited a district hospital targeted in the war, its ward walls still bearing bullet holes and scorch marks. They traveled past makeshift villages formed when hundreds of thousands of Mozambicans returned from refugee camps in Malawi. Most came with little more than UN-issue blue plastic sheets they fashioned into hut roofs and sacks of maize flour bearing a U.S. aid agency's red-white-and-blue logo. "Food and shelter, courtesy of the other world," Glenn jotted in his notebook.

The meeting with Niassa health officials yielded disheartening news: Where a UN-sponsored goiter control project should have been under way, Glenn found only lapsed treatment and empty promises. With no medication to offer, he instead gave a pep talk, focusing on what villagers might do for themselves instead of waiting on some outside savior. "The people in Niassa have been failed," he wrote in his notebook, "and that includes the personnel in the health field who are the real heroes trying to cope with problems."

Frustrated after days encountering people he felt largely powerless to help, Glenn arrived with Ivo in Cuamba, a small town known chiefly as the railhead for train travel into Malawi. Seeing many trains on one side of the tracks and none of them moving, the doctors inquired. Flooding had closed the road to Malawi and undermined the rail bridge. Rebels also claimed to have sabotaged a bridge, but it was unknown which one. Consequently, no trains had moved in a week, though the rail inspector might take a test car out soon.

The doctors proceeded to rounds in Cuamba's district hospital, where staff brought them an urgent case. In the night, a woman in her early twenties had delivered her fourth child. The small baby boy with a sponge of curly hair had a malformed rectum that made it impossible for him to pass waste. If it could not be corrected, the child would not live. The mother spoke only the local dialect, Makua. As she and Glenn tried to speak through translators and with gestures, he addressed her as "Mama" and she called him her one English word: "Okay."

Glenn helped hospital staff run a tube through the baby's nose into his stomach and an IV line in his arm for fluids. An X-ray could have shown

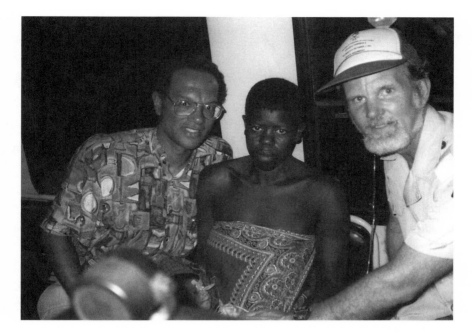

At a small hospital in Cuamba, Mozambique, Glenn and his Mozambiquan colleague Dr. Ivo Garrido met a mother whose newborn needed an operation best performed at a better-equipped hospital hours away. Using the only vehicle available, a railroad maintenance car, Garrido and Glenn made the late-night trip with the baby and the woman Glenn knew only as "the good Mama."

whether the birth defect was something Glenn could fix relatively simply, but the hospital's X-ray machine had long since stopped working. He could try to operate anyway, with hopes of transferring the tiny patient later to a better-equipped hospital. Or, since he and Ivo needed to find a way out of Cuamba themselves, they could take mother and baby with them. As his journal recorded, "That's what we did," hitching a ride with a railway inspector named Oscar.

> *Oscar was willing to transfer us in the zorra, his own private rail-test car, as he went to inspect the bridge footings in question since the flooding. The zorra as first described to me sounded like the*

kind of handcar pumped in turn-of-the century cartoons by prospectors riding the rails. It turned out to be a diesel-fired rail car with half of the platforms holding a derrick and repair equipment, and an enclosed cabin up front. It was headed toward Malawi from Cuamba. For a moment, the prospect of riding backwards for 300 kilometers through a rainstorm struck me as funny if not nauseating. But when told to scramble for a departure, we quickly got ready.

With Ivo supporting Mama and I cradling a thirty-six-hour-old neonate with an IV bottle held high, we prepared for quite an adventure. We situated this stoical, brave woman in the train cabin and supported her feet upon my duffle bag. The hospital sent food for her wrapped up in a swaddling cloth for the transit of we knew not how long and we knew not how far.

Baby has passed neither stool nor urine, unable to do either with a nasogastric drainage tube and IV drip. I was happy that he occasionally burst into lusty gurgling and squirming, which Mama, experienced as she was, responded to invariably by nursing the baby, nasogastric tube notwithstanding. With a spectacular sunset behind us over Malawi, large thunderheads rolling ahead of us, what looked for all the world like Yosemite Valley on either side of us, and rain beginning to spatter the head of the zorra, we rolled out of the station. The zorra was a Noah's Ark of one ailing newborn, one postpartum working Mama, one very nervous chief railway inspector, one Eduardo Mondlane University professor of surgery, and one Fulbright scholar, plus two relatives of the conductor back near the door with three live chickens snatching at corn scattered for their amusement in transit.

Here was a woman who had just given birth, clutching a son who had very limited prospects and faced at least significant surgical treatments. She understood not one word of anything that was being transmitted in a totally foreign environment, and surely had made no trip of this kind before in her life! I smiled and tried to reassure Mama. When she looked concerned about something, I would explain it to her mainly in pantomime to which she would respond with my name, "Okay! Okay!" One of us was a lot braver and much more trusting than the other.

Oscar's task was to test and approve the track so that new diesel locomotives pulling big trains might follow. The older engines that operated on these tracks could pull only six to eight cars, but the newer engines are bigger, more powerful and much faster, pulling twenty cars. People from the bush became used to walking the rails, where the traveling is easier. They learned that when they heard the sounds of an oncoming train, they had time to turn around, look and leisurely walk clear of the rails. The bigger locomotives, though, are much faster and cannot be outrun — but the learning curve is such that anyone who has had the encounter with one of these new engines will not be around to pass along this information. Those who have witnessed the encounters refer to the new locomotive as "Ninjas," because they always kill.

Near the eroded embankment, we slowed to a stop and got out in the rain with my flashlight to check the bridge. Oscar looked with some satisfaction on the new crushed rock that had been piled along the side to divert water and diffuse the weight of the big new trains. As we went over it and backed up, there was no change in this bed of tracks, and he was very pleased. We proceeded on, passing signs that marked villages and train stations. There, poor people who had exhausted their food supply waiting over a week were overjoyed to see an approaching headlight, then dismayed when the zorra slipped past them in the night.

As we rumbled down the rail again, Oscar made increasingly urgent calls into the radio microphone in Portuguese, pleading for an answer, but none returned. When we finally came to the midpoint station, a man outlined only by his own torchlight was standing over the gandy switch, and when we asked why he did not respond, he answered, "Radio no functionando." Of course. This turned out to be of more than casual significance. When Oscar's rail-inspection car had crossed over the bridge and found it safe, that message had gone on to other stations — and one of the Ninjas was coming head-on toward us with no knowledge of where we were.

I joined the rail inspector in straining my eyes as far ahead of the lamp as we could see, looking for any speck of light. We were closing in on the Ninja at half the rate it would be coming toward us. Our only chance was to reach a station about ten kilometers on, which had a side track where we could wait out the passage of the Ninja.

With bells clanging, we reached the station. There was the gandy dancer, scarcely visible in the blackness, but he got the message: After the zorra pulled past, he threw the switch and Oscar guided the test car into the sidetrack. As we came to a stop, Mama had a problem: She needed to pee. So I took "Bebe," and Ivo handed Mama down so that she could squat between the rails. Then he and I exchanged roles as I went to fetch her back up, not an easy task on a black, rainy night.

Then we saw it. It really was fast! By the time we were sure that it was a headlamp, it was almost upon us. Having no warning from the dead radio at the midpoint station, the Ninja surely was surprised to encounter us. As the locomotive swooshed by, I snapped a flash photo, illuminating the faces of the engineers. They could not have looked more startled to see a white man standing in a derrick car in the rain next to a woman being handed a newborn hooked to an IV bottle. Had we still been in shouting distance, I would have called after them: "Why, doesn't this happen all the time?"

Finally, we made it. It was approaching two o'clock as we scrambled across the rail-marshalling yards, carrying baby and helping a blood-dripping Mama up to the platform. The station police were so nonplussed that they didn't even ask us what we were doing, since there didn't seem to be an explanation that would be satisfactory given any amount of imagination.

We got the Hospital Central de Nampula ambulance, a closed truck with benches inside, and the driver had Ivo beside him in front while I took Mama and baby in back. This may well have been the most life-threatening component of our trip. To say that the streets of Nampula have potholes is not quite correct. There is a bit of pavement, just enough to cause disjointing collisions by each wheel *each second at first-gear speed. I was thrown to the floor, and the luggage all overturned, and the water bottles were smashed, and food spilled, but I managed to hang on to the IV bottle, and she still clutched Bebe. She is a good Mama.*

We delivered her—complete with a written transfer note into the casualty ward—saw her into a ward bed, and notified the pediatrician on call. Ivo insisted, "If they need us, they know where to find us; so now, to bed." We checked in to the nearby Hotel Luso, where top-of-the-line suites go for US$18—$2 short of the wage an average Mozambican makes in a month.

In Mozambique with Ivo, Glenn had found a situation he would identify for years to come as the most worthy setting for his missions. He listed the characteristics: "Feeble capacity, extremely limited resources, a very tiny cadre of dedicated people against overwhelming odds." His Mozambican friends had an optimistic Portuguese phrase for such desperate situations: *bastante a começar*, enough to begin. Let other physicians, other Fulbright scholars, choose projects that started closer to the finish line, where obvious success was within easier reach. Glenn preferred the opposite; he preferred to use his skills where there was only, barely, *bastante a começar*.

In early 1997, the *Windmill Herald*, a Dutch-English biweekly newspaper serving North America's Dutch immigrant community, carried a long column of obituary notices. In listings of the deceased and the spouses that survived or predeceased them, most of the names marched two-by-two—"Paul Dykstra, husband of Gertrude;" "Winnie Huizenga, widow of Justus"—but one listing stood apart: "William Geelhoed, widower of Frances, formerly widower of Grace (1985) and Alice (1977); Grand Rapids, MI, Feb. 15, 1997."

Bill Geelhoed died halfway through his ninety-eighth year. Though he had outlasted three wives, he also had lived to see his four children produce twelve grandchildren, who had given him nine great-grandchildren. In Glenn's view, his father had had a long and well-lived life, aiming to learn something new each day, pumping his bicycle around town until a few weeks before his death. From the journal entries and memorials Glenn wrote about his father's death, a single plaintive line stands out: "It is a sad time, as I think that I am now nobody's son."

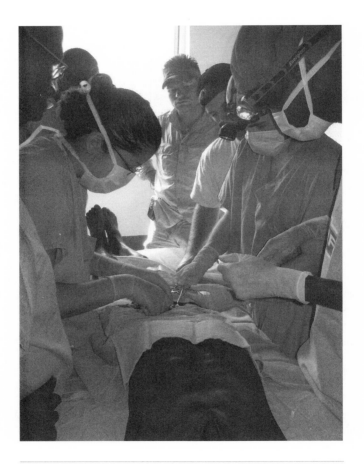

With every mission team, Glenn emphasizes the imperative of sharing knowledge and skills with local practitioners, and providing excellent care even without sophisticated technology. Here, locals and mission team members operate together during a 2009 trip to Duk Payuel, South Sudan.

CHAPTER NINE

The Gift of Deprivation

THE SCIENCE OF EPIDEMIOLOGY IS THE STUDY OF PATTERNS, CAUSES and control of diseases. The practice of epidemiology, Glenn likes to say, is what he does on every mission.

Across continents and populations, on trip after trip, Glenn has seen one pervasive pattern: "haves" and "have-nots," healthy people and sick people—and ironclad correlations of wealth with health, destitution with disease. Mission trips alone cannot change that pattern significantly or permanently. Donated medications run out; volunteer personnel go home.

What Glenn has seen begin to change the equation, in even the most deprived settings, is knowledge. With the clinical information and training that mission teams impart, indigenous practitioners are better able to treat their communities' patients long after the visitors are gone.

That's why on mission trips Glenn aims never to do a procedure unless a local health-care practitioner or trainee is working alongside him. "The skill must be transplanted," he wrote in a journal entry. "Health care is not something to come and push out of the back of the plane like a bag of rice. That's the difference between relief and development. I don't do relief."

Glenn expects mission team members to share skills and expertise with developing-world practitioners. But he reminds them of what he first learned on his own med-school trip to Nigeria, that approaches devised in "medical-center civilization" might not transplant well to the developing world. He asks team members to prepare to practice the ultimate in health-care minimalism, with as little reliance as possible on electricity, plumbing, sophisticated tools and ample supplies, and as much as possible on medical basics and ingenuity.

Glenn also warns team members that their living conditions will be as impoverished as the clinical setting: meager diets, bare-bones lodging, few creature comforts. He can tell them what to pack to make "roughing it" a little less rough—energy bars and powdered Gatorade, bath-in-a-bag towelettes. But he has no use for volunteers who complain about a few days of deprivation when those around them have known nothing else—people who, as he once wrote, "want a rip-roaring adventure but, at the end of the day, expect a cold beer and hot shower." Before each trip launches, Glenn tries to weed out such applicants with a bracing, three-part statement of his mission priorities:

Your survival is my obligation.

Your health and safety are my concerns.

Your comfort doesn't even make it to my radar screen
ahead of these people we are going there to help.

Glenn knows the statement sounds harsh. But he wants prospective team members to think clearly about what they'll face, and that isn't always the case when their hearts are set on going. Many of them describe the same, powerful motivation: *I've received so much in my life; now I want to give back.* It's a noble thought Glenn never would discourage—as an ideal. But in reality, he has learned, even the most well-intentioned volunteers may find it harder than they had imagined to serve in deprived settings.

From a mission trip to Haiti, Glenn's journal recalls an exchange with a twenty-one-year-old medical student, "a pretty young woman with all the right fingernails and eyelashes. At one point she announced, 'I need dessert.' I observed that she was quite possibly the first person I ever had heard describe dessert as a need. But I counseled her not to worry, and I gestured toward a patient, rail-thin and wearing probably the only clothes he owned. 'See that man over there? If you need dessert, perhaps you can go get his.' She seemed to get my meaning."

By the end of the mission, the student's view of her needs and the world's had shifted. Before the trip, she told Glenn, "I was a spoiled brat." After the trip, she was no less privileged, but she was personally, painfully aware of how many on the planet are not.

Glenn's chief goal for missions is to have positive, lasting effects for patients, to help as many as possible while there and to embed knowledge that will help more in the future. But he also knows that invariably the patients will have a profound effect on his team members. He calls this witnessing of how people adapt, survive and even thrive in the face of chronic deprivation one of the most valuable "gifts from the poor" that he and teammates derive. "These people face larger numbers of bigger problems with far fewer resources than you or I ever will," he says. "We have so much to learn from them!"

The lesson can be a brutal one. Face-to-face with people whose unmet needs are staggering, some team members despair and break down. When that happens Glenn takes them on "walkabout" to discuss what they're experiencing. Many express the same anguish: "This is impossible!" "I can't do enough!" "There are a hundred problems I can't fix!"

Glenn hears them out. Then he encourages them to begin again with something —anything—that contributes, even if it's just hanging hospital linens to dry. "We do what we can do with what we have," he counsels. Then he recounts his own experience of learning this lesson while on a mission in one of the poorest countries on earth. His journal entry calls it "my Swaziland story."

Raleigh Fitkin Memorial Hospital, in the central Swaziland city of Manzini. I look around and see thirty people lying in bed with one of their legs "in traction." For the lower extremity, we have but one goal: ten toes headed in the same direction on limbs of equal length. How do you achieve that when leg bones are fractured? In the developed world, we might operate to set bones or insert rods. But this is a poor country, and this is the tropics, where doing anything invasive risks infection. So patients are put in traction.

This means getting a rope, taping one end to their skin, tying the other end to a coffee can filled with sand, and that's supposed to be pulling their leg straight. Well, that hurts, so they're going to do something to foil the system 100 percent of the time — put a brick under the can or shift in bed. Some of these people have been here for months to years. What incentive is there to leave when they're being fed three meals a day? But their injuries are not healing.

A patient comes in with his thigh bone broken straight through. He had slipped in rainy-season mud and fallen down a river bank. This grizzled old orderly brings me the X-ray; he doesn't speak English well, but he is listening all the time. There's nobody around to consult, so here I am, holding the X-ray up to the window and talking to myself: "This would be an ideal patient for internal fixation; we could put a rod right through the middle of the bone and have the guy up and around within the day. But under the circumstances, considering where we are, we will hang him up in traction."

I am confident I've gone through the options, discussed with the air what should be done under ideal circumstances and what will be done here for practical reasons. Then I feel a tug on my sleeve. It's the grizzled old man, and he's gesturing to me to come with him. He brings me to the courtyard and points at two kids, the most grotesque little hominids you've ever seen. Completely ruined, lying there, virtually no function in their limbs, they're wards of the hospital and get fed whatever is left over.

This orderly points to them and says to me, "You weren't here. You weren't here." And then he points to the X-ray of the broken femur and says, "You are here."

Talk about lessons for living. I say to him, "Of course, you're right." I walk back and find Beauty, the hospital matron. I say, "Beauty, let me see your orthopedic-surgery instruments." She takes me back to the supply room and she proudly brings out this shrouded case with dust on it. We open it up, and there's a carpenter's brace and bit, a hammer, and a chisel. Everyone on staff is looking at me. I look at Beauty, I look at the tools, and I say out loud, "Matron, these instruments are forty years out of date!" Everyone stares at the spoiled American brat. And I look around sheepishly and say, "Hey, forty years out of date—that's me!"

We did the internal-fixation operation, stuffed a rod in the man's leg, and put a splint on him to stabilize it. And the following day he was ambulatory in the ward. The staff says to me, "You'd better go to the operating room." Why? Because about twenty-five of those thirty people who've been lying in traction all these months are saying, "I want this operation!"

So here's my conclusion. I am not an orthopedist. But compared to what? I did not have the best tools, but I had something. I could have told the patient, "Go to the hospital in Johannesburg," but I *might as well have told him there's a good hospital on the second ring of Saturn. I was the only person there who might help, so I fixed what I could fix.*

The discussions were lengthy and intense, and the central question was roughly this: We see so much human suffering in the world and we seek ways to alleviate it, but by what measure will we know whether we succeed?

Glenn remembers noting the irony of well-dressed, well-fed men discussing how to heal a suffering planet, over lunch at the Cosmos Club. The "clubhouse" that is Cosmos Club headquarters is an elegant French Renaissance mansion on the prime Washington, D.C., real estate known as Embassy Row. The Cosmos Club society was founded in 1878 by distinguished figures in science, literature and the arts, including John Wesley Powell, a geologist and Grand Canyon explorer. Powell sought a setting where leading thinkers "could meet socially and exchange ideas, where vitality would grow from the mixture of disciplines." The elected-members-only club became a locus for America's political and intellectual elite; members over the years have included three U.S. presidents and two vice presidents, a dozen Supreme Court justices and thirty-two Nobel Prize winners.

The quarterly lunches Glenn attended in the early 1990s were convened by scholar and author Ralph G. H. Siu. A pioneer in synthesizing differing cultures, Siu proposed a new academic discipline to study the infliction of human suffering by individuals, corporations, governments and other institutions. Siu called the discipline panetics, after a term from the Pali language of Buddha: *paneti*, "to inflict." Through his International Society for Panetics (ISP), Siu hoped to foster a consensus approach to reducing the suffering humans inflict on each other.

Glenn had seen brutal examples of that, on missions to tribal lands where warring factions attacked, sacked and starved each other. With Siu, Glenn and other ISP scholars explored both broader and subtler situations in which

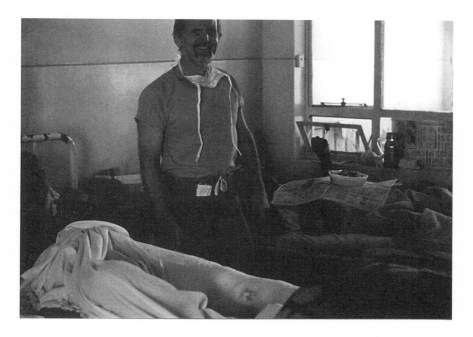

At Raleigh Fitkin Memorial Hospital in Manzini, Swaziland, Glenn found numerous patients who had been consigned to traction because of broken leg bones. His ability to operate successfully on many of them, even with outdated instruments in an impoverished setting, taught him a lesson about what he calls "the gift of deprivation."

pain might be inflicted. How much suffering is caused by, or relieved by, U.S. defense spending? Health-care programs? Unregulated business practices?

Taking the measure of suffering was something Glenn and fellow physicians did with patients all the time: How bad is the pain? What makes it better or worse? In the same vein, ISP created a measurable unit of human-inflicted suffering. Siu called it the *dukkha*, from the Pali word for pain. On a one-to-nine scale, one *dukkha* was equivalent to one day of a tolerable toothache, while nine *dukkhas* was pain of such unbearable intensity that the sufferer wanted to die. Quantity of suffering was calculated by multiplying the intensity of suffering by the duration in days.

Siu used the *dukkha* less as a way to very precisely measure pain than as a tool to provoke debate and research. The important thing, he contended, was to establish freedom from infliction of suffering as a human right, and then to focus public and private policy on eliminating it.

Glenn considered panetics an intriguing approach. If suffering could reliably be measured, so could the success of efforts to alleviate it—his efforts and others'. The scientist in him liked having metrics; the humanitarian in him loved solving people's problems. Glenn served as an ISP officer and wrote and presented papers for society gatherings. After Siu's death, in 1998, Glenn helped arrange the archiving of Siu's papers so that researchers could access them. But ultimately Glenn could linger only so long over quantifying human suffering before he was back to his preferred pursuit: treating it.

On mission trips to northern India, southern Sudan and Malawi, then-GWU medical student John Sutter was struck by "one thing Glenn does: He sets an example for experiencing hardship. We were in the Himalayas, and at one point our jeeps got stuck in a creek we tried to cross. We all got out and pushed, and in the process he rolled his ankle and ended up fracturing his foot. He basically laced up his boot tighter for the rest of the trip, another week and a half.

"On many of these trips, the situations we're working with are, for all intents and purposes, immense suffering, intense health problems and poverty. Occasionally somebody on a trip—who maybe didn't go through the screening process as honestly as they should have—will end up complaining about accommodations or worrying about where to take a shower. But Glenn, by example, doesn't complain about anything. He wants for nothing."

What patients teach Glenn about persevering despite deprivation, Glenn then helps team members learn, Sutter says. His summary of that lesson: "If you have your basic health and you're taking in almost enough calories every day, then everything else is gravy.

"In the Sudan we slept under mosquito nets in 110-degree heat. We ate one meal a day, and we didn't have enough water. But the people we were

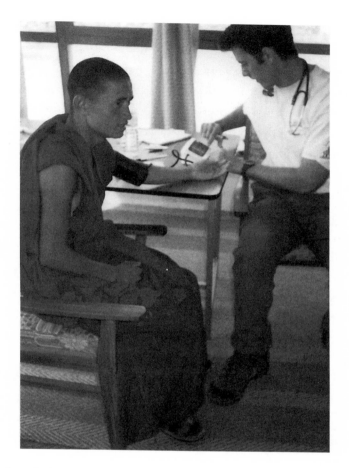

While studying for his medical degree, onetime paramedic John Sutter went on several medical missions with Glenn. In Ladakh in northern India, his patient caseload included monks from a nearby monastery.

treating were going through a lot more than we were.

"It was a humbling experience. I've always sort of had my priorities straight: trying to be a good person, not being materialistic, giving back. But on these trips, those types of values are solidified. In southern Sudan we worked with people who were very, very sick and with little or no means for health care and betterment, and every once in a while northern forces were taking gunships down the Nile and strafing these people's villages. How do you see that and then come back home and complain if your computer is on the fritz or the subway is crowded?"

When Bill Barrett was a surgical resident at GWU, he also joined Glenn on a northern India mission. Now Dr. Barrett is an acute-care and trauma surgeon who has treated impoverished patients from the Indian reservations of the American southwest to South America and Africa. "Like Glenn, I have a passion for providing my services to people who need them the most," Barrett says. He credits Glenn for helping him acquire the skills and judgment to provide excellent care even in resource-deprived settings. And he calls Glenn "a modern-day surgical philosopher" who has influenced his view of the next frontier in healing.

Over the past forty years, Barrett says, "most of the advances in surgery were technological advances, new techniques" like the trailblazing transplant operations of Glenn's Harvard years. The next forty years, he believes, "will be about how to take all this technology and this level of care and provide it for those who really need it, instead of just in the United States and other developed countries.

"There are, what, more than six billion people on this planet? And I'd say one billion of them have access to really good medical care, but the rest probably do not. That's where the advances are going to be made in the next forty years, in distribution. And Glenn went from being an academician, doing research and writing papers, to going around the world and figuring out how to take surgery and widen its distribution.

"Glenn got into general surgery because it was the specialty where you got all the toughest cases and the sickest people, and it was a challenge. I can see why Glenn was attracted to that. Back in the day when ground was being broken with new techniques and limits were being pushed from a technical standpoint, that was the place for him. But when it became a matter of surgical colleagues fighting with each other over who got to do the next hernia repair, I don't think he was interested in that at all. So it became, 'If there are no more big operations to be developed, now I want to go on a different adventure: How can I operate with a knife and fork in the back of a pickup truck in a war zone?' That's the kind of guy he is."

Stepping into the lives of the world's poorest patients gives not one gift but several, Glenn has learned. Mission team members return with new survival skills, both practical and psychological. Sharply reminded of their blessings, many recommit to what Glenn calls "leaning more lightly on the planet"—wasting and consuming less, conserving and appreciating more. Most important, once team members have so intimately encountered these global problems, they feel obliged to help create solutions. It's just the reaction Glenn hopes for and wrote about in a brief reflection he titled "Activate the Geezer":

> *Throughout my tours of Africa or other areas of the former British Empire, I would periodically hear a suggestion that I "activate the geezer." When I have occasion to run or climb or explore jungles, I have one particular need upon return, and that is for hot water, preferably in a shower or bucket bath. To obtain it, you have to "activate the geezer"—a unit that has been called a "geiser" in other parts of the world, and in America is known as a hot water heater.*
>
> *"Activate the geezer." Though I laugh each time I hear it, I choose to take this advice to heart in another way. I consider activating the geezer fine marching orders for those of us who have become complacent in our comfortable environments. Turning the tap produces a stream of hot water only in certain very privileged areas of the world. What we need to do is to be activated ourselves in order to make such improvements possible for others.*

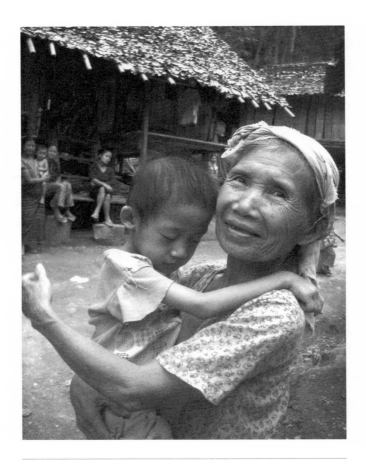

A passage from one of Glenn's favorite quotations—"How far you go in life depends on your being tender with the young (and) compassionate with the aged"—fit the clientele he found on a 2010 medical mission to internally displaced persons in Myanmar (also known as Burma).

Chapter Ten

From Suffering, the Gift of Strength

"HOW FAR YOU GO IN LIFE DEPENDS ON YOUR BEING TENDER WITH THE young, compassionate with the aged, sympathetic with the striving, and tolerant of the weak and the strong, because someday in life you will have been all of these."

This saying, attributed to pioneering scientist George Washington Carver, is one of Glenn's favorites. He finds many opportunities to slip it into conversation because it describes, in essence, his chosen clientele. The young, the aged and the striving all are embraced by his far-flung practice. So are the weak and the strong, but on those traits Glenn sees his developing-world patients differently than others might.

"When most Westerners look at the world's poorest people, they see suffering as the defining characteristic," he once wrote. "They see the suffering but not the adaptation, the courage, the intelligence—the strength."

On every mission, Glenn meets exemplars of strength despite suffering, ordinary individuals with an extraordinary ability to thrive despite crushing burdens. He has coined an admiring term for them: "subcultural giants." He delights in learning about their lives and sharing their stories with colleagues. And he is especially pleased when the giants, by their example, spur his mission members to summon unexpected strengths of their own.

The daughter of archaeologists, Elizabeth Yellen spent much of her child-hood in Africa and has always felt at home in the developing world. She went to high school in Washington, D.C., and college at Harvard, rowing on a national-championship team and exploring various career paths. "I was one of those people who liked everything," she recalls, "but I loved medicine, how it brought everything together. It felt useful and essential, important to all people everywhere."

After a stint in Appalachia working on health care for the rural poor, Yellen entered GWU medical school. She knew Glenn not only as a professor but as a student: Her mother was Glenn's thesis adviser when he earned his master's degree in anthropology. On the eve of her third year of med school, Yellen joined Bill Barrett on Glenn's medical-mission-plus-Himalayan-hiking-trek to the Ladakh region, in the Tibetan plateau of northern Indian.

Yellen remembers the arrival in Ladakh for its mountain vistas—"like something out of *National Geographic*"—and for the altitude sickness she felt at nearly three miles above sea level. After two days, she had acclimated enough to join Glenn for an early morning run through the stunning scenery. "It was one of those moments where you have an 'Is this real?' thought, and that's kind of a metaphor for my missions with Glenn," she says now. "You follow him and trust him and get into crazy situations, and it ends up being an amazing experience."

In most U.S. medical schools, students spend the first two years getting classroom training, not clinical experience. Yellen had never done patient care before the Ladakh mission. Now, she and the rest of Glenn's team would spend fourteen days in dawn-to-dusk clinics, seeing several hundred patients a day. "At first," she recalls, "I felt like, 'What am I doing? How can I be treating patients?'"

In a remote hill station called Manali, Yellen met two practitioners who once were as inexperienced as she, Dr. Laji Varghese and his wife, Dr. Sheila. The couple fell in love while students at a Christian medical school in Punjab. He trained in internal medicine, she in ob-gyn. After graduation, both felt their faith called them to serve where the need was great.

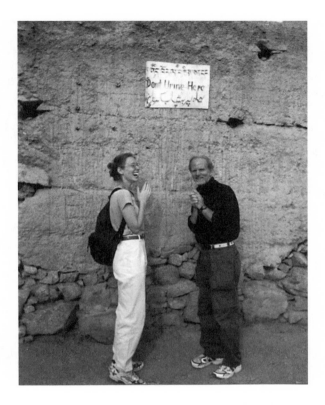

On a mission to Ladakh in northern India, medical student Elizabeth Yellen and Glenn mug for the camera under a sign warning, "Don't Urine Here."

Manali fit that description. The Vargheses had heard it called "the end of the habitable world." Winters were cruel, laborers lived on less than a dollar a day, and government health care was hours away, even if patients could afford it. In the 1930s, an English noblewoman had established a small charity dispensary in Manali, but the Lady Willingdon Hospital had had no doctor on staff for a year, until June 1979, when Laji and Sheila arrived, newly married. They had only basic MD training, no background in hospital administration, and no money; the hospital had very little equipment, no running water and erratic electricity.

The Vargheses imagined the posting would last a year. More than thirty years later, it remains their life's work.

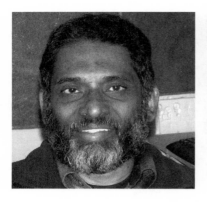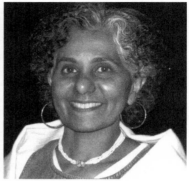

Photos: Sheila Varghese

Though Dr. Laji Varghese and his wife, Dr. Sheila Varghese, had heard Manali in northern India called "the end of the habitable world," they went there fresh out of medical school to staff a small hospital. More than 30 years later, they still are there, shepherding a hospital and remote clinics that care for tens of thousands of patients every year.

"I was so awed talking to them," Yellen recalls. "They sought out this underserved population and then realized they needed many more specialized skills than they had trained in. So they really taught themselves to do everything," by learning new techniques from the doctors who came for medical missions.

Glenn vividly recalls scenes from his collaborations with the unstoppable couple: Laji powering through one operation after another—club feet, hysterectomies, gallbladder removals—in "scrubs" he made by sterilizing cloth sleeves in a pressure cooker and then fastening them over his street clothes; Sheila, gracious and soft-spoken, quickly jumping into action in obstetric emergencies, instilling confidence in the frightened midwives; Laji in a dim, makeshift clinic, operating by the light of a mountain climber's headlamp that Glenn has used on missions ever since.

Through the years, Laji and Sheila helped establish a school and then an orphanage in Manali. In villages one hundred to two hundred kilometers away, they founded rural clinics staffed by health workers they trained. Though Lady Willingdon Hospital never has had more than fifty beds, it has admitted as many as 3,000 patients a year and served twelve times more as outpatients.

Yellen and Barrett found the Vargheses every bit as inspiring as Glenn had promised they would be. Working with Laji, Glenn and others on the Ladakh mission team, Yellen learned procedures, gained experience and had a revelation. "I realized I did have tools," she recalls. "And even if they were small tools, for people who had no contact with medical care and no other opportunity, those tools could be huge.

"I went on the trip primarily to give back to people I thought might not get care otherwise, but I got so much out of it for myself. I learned the value of thinking beyond whatever category you've got yourself in: How can I really be useful, what's really the need I want to answer, and how do I do that?"

Yellen changed her return ticket to stay and work in Manali for two more weeks. Barrett ended up staying three months to work in Ladakh and especially with Laji, whom he calls "just an unbelievable surgeon. He never went through a residency; he basically trained himself. Yet the number of operations he does in a day is probably three to four times what American surgeons average, because the room turnover is faster. He has come up with lots of efficiencies; we were usually done with surgery at 3:00 p.m. and playing badminton at 4:00 p.m.

"In the United States, we have figured out how to make medical care very expensive, and there are a million reasons for that," Barrett says. "But it can be done just as well for one-twentieth of the cost, and that's been proven" by mission-field doctors like Laji, Sheila and Glenn.

When Glenn e-mailed the Vargheses his year-end letter in 2009, he asked for an update on their work. Laji wrote right back, wishing Glenn a Christmas season of "peace and rest" but describing little of the latter in his own life. He and Sheila had stepped down from directing Lady Willingdon to divide their time between the hospital's satellite clinics, Manali's school and medical missions of their own, including one to Uganda.

"It's fun, but tiring and challenging," Laji wrote to Glenn. "I would love to travel with you someday and help train young doctors who like this kind of life." His update ended with a list of questions: Did Glenn know anyone who might send him sutures and needles? Who might cover school fees for five students at his orphanage? Who might "want to be involved long term" at Lady Willingdon?

Glenn forwarded Laji's wish list to prospective donors and looked through his stockpiles of mission supplies for suture materials. Then he wrote to the Medical Mission Hall of Fame Foundation, suggesting that the Vargheses be considered for induction. In his estimation, they are the kinds of heroes who should be recognized as well as emulated: dedicated professionals who, out of very little, have made a huge difference in many lives.

In the southern African nation of Malawi, one in four children do not live to the age of five. Of Malawians who reach adulthood, one in eight carries the AIDS virus; life expectancy is roughly forty-one years.

In north-central Malawi, close to the border with Zambia, lies Embangweni, a town of some five thousand souls. In 1902, two Scottish missionaries—physician Agnes Fraser and her preacher-husband, Donald—established the outpost called Loudon Mission Station and the health-care dispensary that today is Embangweni Hospital. The 130-bed hospital and its four satellite clinics serve a population of more than 100,000 people.

For years Embangweni Hospital's permanent staff included just one physician, American-born Dr. Martha Sommers, who also worked part-time at a hospital farther north. Most care is provided by clinical officers who have taken three years of classes and served a year's internship, or by medical assistants with even less training. So the hospital staff welcomes the extra hands of medical mission teams, like the ones Glenn has led to Embangweni five times since 1999.

Glenn and team members invariably return from Embangweni with tales of the courage and resilience they witnessed: from pupils at a school for the hearing-impaired, from patients in the AIDS and maternity wards, and from a veteran hospital staffer known to all as Mr. Tembo.

Sommers calls Mr. Tembo "the best surgical assistant you will ever find." Glenn, borrowing a term from social change theory, calls Mr. Tembo a "positive deviant"—that exceptional individual who, with the same resources as those around him, achieves markedly better results.

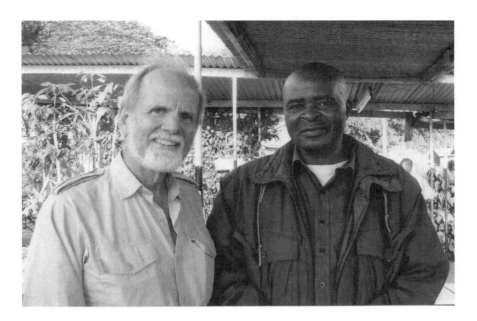

On missions to Embangweni Hospital in Malawi, Glenn worked repeatedly with a medical orderly known to all as "Mr. Tembo." Though not formally educated, Mr. Tembo is, in Glenn's view, as skilled and experienced at some procedures as many of the surgeons he assists.

In the 1950s, Wyson Tembo was among the 90 percent of Malawi's children with no chance to attend secondary school. But as Glenn wrote of Tembo in an essay, "he did not want to be limited by this education so set about attempting to help in any way that he could. He applied to and achieved a position in the hospital whereby he could assist, in whatever way he might be able, in the daily workings in the operating theater. Before long, he was not only the jack of all trades, but had initiated several programs in which the trade could actually be done more smoothly and with fewer resources."

First Mr. Tembo observed the surgeons. Then he assisted them, working with many who, like Glenn, were eminent practitioners and teachers in their home countries. Though by official job title Mr. Tembo remains essentially a medical orderly, Glenn considers him as experienced and skilled at some procedures as many of the surgeons he assists.

Elizabeth Yellen worked with Mr. Tembo during a 2002 mission at

Embangweni. "Here's someone who just made something out of nothing, who had no reason to succeed and yet became really the heart and soul of the hospital," she says of the quiet, distinguished-looking man. "He treated people, he triaged people, he guided the visiting doctors who were there through every procedure. You'd see these big British doctors who really were lost in that setting, and he was teaching them how to do C-sections."

In Malawi as in much of sub-Saharan Africa, maternal death rates are among the highest in the world. When women, especially young ones, are incapable of normal delivery, days of unsuccessful labor can end in death. If they can get to Embangweni, both mother and baby often can be saved with a caesarean section. Sommers, who has known Mr. Tembo since 1993, figures he may have assisted with as many as two thousand of the life-saving operations.

By the time of Glenn's 2009 mission to Embangweni, Mr. Tembo was in his sixties, trying without success to retire but getting called back month after month to work at the hospital. "He's amazing at finding that bleeder and helping you stop it. That's where he's at his best; he's an exceptionally great surgical assistant," says Sommers, who in late 2009 transferred to another hospital, leaving Embangweni with no resident doctor.

Seeing Glenn and his team work with Mr. Tembo and the Embangweni staff, Sommers was struck by how Glenn "is so encouraging to everyone, to his people who he brings on missions and to our people who he works with here. He's fun, he's energetic, and," she adds with a laugh, "he also is a good surgeon, because if he wasn't, Mr. Tembo would tell me!" When Glenn's mission team finished its tour and celebrated with an overnight trip to a game park, Glenn took Mr. Tembo along as his guest.

After medical school, Elizabeth Yellen did a pediatrics residency and a cardiology fellowship at Children's Hospital Boston, which is affiliated with Harvard. One lasting impact of her work with Glenn, she says, is that "when I was looking for a job, I really did feel it was important to serve people who might not otherwise be well-served and do as excellent a job as you can for those people, who may never notice what your credentials are." She joined the cardiology staff at Boston Medical Center specifically because that hospital serves low-income and immigrant populations. "I find it really important to do this kind of work," she says. "That was reinforced by the experiences with Doctor G."

Vanessa Goldenberg's decision to enter medicine was shaped by strong women: the visionary doctor she worked for at Duke University Hospital's Breast Wellness Clinic, and the courageous patients she met there, facing down breast cancer.

Just weeks after finishing her first year of medical school at the University of Colorado, Goldenberg was at Embangweni, rotating with Glenn through the surgery, maternity, pediatrics and adult patient wards. With some women patients in particular, she recalls, "Dr. Glenn encouraged me to really look at them and take it all in." He told her she would never forget what she saw: the hardship and suffering, but also the strength and joy.

I delivered my first baby—that was really exciting! An eighteen-year-old woman was having contractions, and when I looked over she was squatting on the bed and the baby's head was coming out. I screamed for the midwife and she said, 'Put on your gloves and you do it.' She kind of talked me through it; she was telling me what to do. The baby was in the exactly perfect position; there were no complications. It was her first baby, and it was a girl. I asked them what the baby's name was, and they told me they don't give the baby the name at birth; they wait a week and then go to the husband's family, which decides the name . . .

The whole experience of being in the maternity ward was really crazy. The women provided the fabric to wrap their babies in. I think the only thing the hospital gave the women was a black, plastic garbage bag that they laid on, on the bed. After they gave birth, they had to get up and clean up all their own fluids and then walk themselves back to bed. And they had twelve hours before they had to leave because the turnover is so high.

The adult female ward was one of the more emotional experiences for me. I became quite close to one patient in particular, Mabel. She was thirty-six years old, a mother of two little girls and a geography teacher in Zambia. She talked to me about her students, how most of them are poor, the hardships they endure, and how much she cared for them. She came in because of pain in her right upper thigh that was so bad she could hardly walk.

Glenn identified a muscle abscess in Mabel's leg. He drained it and showed Goldenberg how to do daily dressing changes. Goldenberg found a crutch and helped Mabel begin walking again. Knowing that such abscesses often are associated with immune system deficiencies, Glenn suggested an HIV test. Mabel agreed. The test came back positive.

"I got there literally seconds after they had told her," Goldenberg recalls. "She was mainly concerned with her children, but she said she had been tested at the time of delivery and that the test was negative. I tried to explain to her that she needed to get on top of getting antiretroviral drugs and treatment for the HIV. One of the clinical officers told me Mabel didn't want to discuss it with her husband. I got the impression she wouldn't be telling anyone in her family. I hope her children aren't HIV-positive.

"I had never seen an AIDS patient before Embangweni. I remember standing in front of these women, finding it difficult not to get emotional. There were several who passed away while we were there. Dr. Glenn had told us to look at them and understand the look in their eyes."

The Swahili word for AIDS is *ukimwi*; the belt in southern Africa where HIV and AIDS are most prevalent has been called the Ukimwi Road. Glenn has spent more than enough time on that road to recognize those nearing its end. His Embangweni journal entries describe three of those patients: One young woman with telltale lesions of Kaposi's sarcoma, too ill to eat or drink; two other women in their mid-thirties, in beds side by side, "each staring blankly into the Valley of the Shadow of Death.

"Their names are Beauty and Fairness. Beauty is thirty-four years old. She has a very kind guardian sitting behind her in bed, propping up her head. She is a woman who may have been pretty perhaps weeks ago. She is unresponsive, staring into my eyes from a very great distance away. She is sitting next to Fairness, who looks so similar—with thin, stick-figure arms—that they could be sisters. I told the students to get to know them quickly and watch the progression of this disease, since they would not likely be here long." Glenn also told the students to watch out the hospital windows for "the equivalent of the angel of death": the oxcarts arriving daily to carry corpses to burial.

The next day, the students brought Glenn the news. Fairness' family had taken her home to die. Beauty had slipped into unconsciousness. And the young woman with Kaposi's sarcoma was gone, borne away on an oxcart as mourners walked alongside. In Embangweni's women's ward, matrons were settling new patients into the remade beds, murmuring words of comfort.

In the poor, hungry, rural villages of northern Malawi, children's lives are uniformly hard. But some children bear an added burden: deafness or severe hearing loss, often from infections that went untreated. From as far as four hundred kilometers away, these children come to live at the region's lone facility for them, the Embangweni School for the Hard of Hearing. During missions to Embangweni, Glenn always takes his teams to the school, where they give students exams and, in return, receive a humbling gift.

The school opened in 1994 with twenty-three students, four teachers and $4,000 in seed money from Marion Medical Mission, an Illinois-based charity. When Marion volunteer Jocelyn Logan met the first students, who had spent years in their home villages isolated and uneducated, she had to teach them how to hold a crayon. Today, the school serves about 180 students in a four-year preschool, eight-year primary school and vocational high school. Youngsters are taught lipreading, oral speech and sign language, in English as well as the national language Chichewa and the local language Chitumbuka.

They study standard subjects and learn basic life skills, raising gardens and farm animals, making furniture, molding bricks for new school buildings.

When Glenn's teams visit, they conduct ear clinics and hearing tests. With intensive cleanings and medications for infections, some youngsters' hearing can be measurably improved. "It was great," says Clare Marcot, a twenty-year-old aspiring teacher on Glenn's 2009 mission team. "The kids were so fantastic, and they loved having us there."

As a thank-you, the students brought out a cherished possession Logan first gave them more than a decade ago: a set of colored handbells with color-coded sheet music. Even those who can't hear a note can feel the vibrations from the resonating bells, and shake them in time with the conductor. They learn every melody as written and then add variations of their own, Logan says. The bell ringers play at school chapel services and, when they can afford transportation, perform concerts in the community.

With a fond chuckle, Marcot describes the bell choir as "very, very loud, for sure, but really good." Glenn, too, has left concerts with his ears ringing— but also with his heart full, at the triumph of the spirit in which joy drowns out affliction.

Through the early and mid-1990s, Glenn made return trips to Assa to continue working on the Goiter Project. On every trip he ferried in as much medical equipment and supplies as the Cessna's weight limit allowed. The Democratic Republic of Congo, always a desperately poor nation, increasingly was also a very dangerous one. Ethnic violence from the Hutu-Tutsi conflict spilled over the border with Rwanda; rebels with the brutal Lord's Resistance Army raided across the border with Uganda. Waves of coups and countercoups meant that on any given day, Assa's residents might be menaced by either regular government troops or renegades.

Glenn's journals noted that the villagers still managed to "do what they do far better than we: dealing with far bigger problems in larger numbers with fewer resources." But after escalating violence in 1995, when Assa's school was totally destroyed and many homes burned, missionaries stationed there had to withdraw. If foreigners' presence had afforded any measure of protection, their departure eliminated it, and Glenn worried about Assa's residents: "Many of them are friends of mine," he wrote, "and they are all my patients."

On the eve of Glenn's return to Assa in early July 1998, he recorded the bad news: "Last week, Assa was stripped bare by a marauding renegade band of troops . . . My friends in Assa fled into the bush. The troops ordered the local chief to dig his own grave, but he escaped when the mavericks got distracted."

Determined not to lose all they had built, the villagers of Assa, as they fled into the bush, carried clinic property with them. Mawa, who worked as a nurse, carried off operating-room equipment and medicines. Fearing for their own property and lives, the villagers still squirreled away the clinic property, guarded it during their exile, and triumphantly brought it back when it was safe to return.

But not all did return. When Glenn reached Assa, he asked after those he did not see. Where was Mawa? Where was the old cook, who had survived generations of civil war? Through a translator, a village leader answered Glenn this way:

We are so happy to see you again and to know that you have returned from so far away, that you and others are still thinking of us. Our hearts are overflowing despite many troubles . . . It is true what you heard, that we were attacked again, and that what little we had was taken away, and that several of us were killed. But to repeat their names and these stories so soon would be to relive the awful events . . . and we are here instead to rejoice with you and with God who has spared us to see you again.

Welcome to Assa, therefore. May we all be so grateful that we can hold back the telling of our troubles and glory instead that we are here and alive together, to start over again."

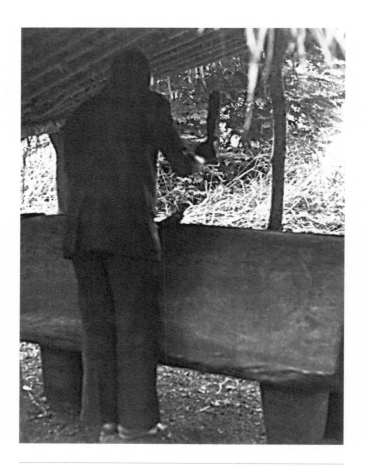

One of Glenn's most treasured keepsakes from repeat missions to Assa, Congo, is a little wooden drum, a replica of the large "talking drum" used to relay drumbeat messages among surrounding villages. The master drummer who made Glenn the gift, Bule, demonstrated that when the big drum nearby was struck, the small one also vibrated—a symbol, Glenn wrote, of "the resonance between me and the people of Assa."

Chapter Eleven

Cultures, Consonants and Vowels

His name does not fit him. When he was a young man working in the Congolese gold fields, someone—perhaps as a joke—called him Bule, which in Swahili means "useless." And Bule he has remained, despite his many useful pursuits: blacksmith, herbalist, preacher, jack-of-all-trades.

When Christian missionaries established a station in Assa that shortwave radio signals could not reach, one indispensable person they brought with them was Bule. It was he who created and maintains a vital tool for communication, the "talking drum."

With an artistry passed from his father's father, Bule fashioned a hollow log into a cylindrical, footed drum eight feet long. In the drum's top he carved a slit. He thinned the drum wall on one side of the slit and left it thicker on the other, giving the instrument two distinct tones. With short wooden drumsticks coated in rubbery tree resin, he beats out rhythmic patterns of high and low tones—messages that can be heard for great distances, in a code he and other drummers (and most of Zandeland's elders) understand.

When signals from Bule's "master" drum are heard in the next village, a drummer repeats them on his "messenger" drum. Those signals are heard in the next village and replayed on the next drum, then the next, in scores of relays that cover hundreds of kilometers. It is said that the relayed message can be heard all the way to the capital, Kinshasa, though few there hear and recognize it over the din of their radios and phones. While growing swaths of Africa possess twenty-first-century communications tools, Zandeland still counts on the drummers for important local news.

Every time Glenn visited Assa, villagers who had virtually nothing still found gifts to give as a welcome. A family whose hut Glenn passed while he was heading out for a run had picked and prepared two ripe pineapples by the time he ran back. An old hunter brought him a small clutch of eggs, which was quite a bit more protein than the old man had consumed that week, Glenn felt certain. Others gave firewood, bananas, rice.

Bule's gift was a carving: a miniature version of the master drum, with miniature sticks for beating it.

As Glenn cradled the toy drum admiringly, Bule tugged him over to the thatched-roof shelter that houses the master drum. Bule raised his arms, closed his eyes, and brought the sticks down on the drum. A few beats into the rhythm, Bule abruptly stopped, muffling the master drum with both hands. Still, a low tone lingered. Glenn thought it was the sound of a distant relay drum—until Bule came to him and touched the miniature drum, and the low tone vanished. Bule repeated the demonstration, to be sure Glenn understood.

"The profound meaning of his gift moved me," Glenn wrote in his journal. "Wherever I may be, there will always be a resonance between me and the people of Assa." On missions, this is what Glenn seeks for himself and his traveling companions: the privilege of entering a culture on the terms of its inhabitants.

The anthropologist in Glenn is mindful of what he calls "the fundamental modification of the observed: that any time you study something, you change it." He plans missions expressly to effect some changes—to heal the sick and to train indigenous healers. Beyond that, he tries to live as the locals live, to follow their cultural scripts, to leave populations largely as he found them. He asks team members to adopt the same approach, and he offers two ground rules:

(1) *Resist the impulse, however well-meaning,
to try to change the host culture.*

(2) *Embrace how the host culture may change you,
if your heart and mind are open.*

Glenn cautions his recruits about the pitfalls of what he calls "white-people-off-the-airplane medicine." That's his description of foreign medical teams that drop in briefly to provide treatment but no training, leaving locals as incapable of caring for themselves as they were before. It's also his short-hand for a mentality that promotes Western-style, one-size-fits-all solutions in settings where they are neither suitable nor sustainable.

Long before he completed a master's degree in anthropology in 1994, Glenn was practicing his own brand of medical anthropology. On missions to every continent, he does not just see patients, he sees patients in context—factoring in genetic and social inheritance, background and mindset, religion, superstition, socialization. If physicians mean their vow to "do no harm," he reasons, they must take time to learn exactly what's deemed harmful and helpful in each population they touch.

In 2007, an obstetrics-gynecology colleague on a mission with Glenn to Sudan came prepared to teach family planning to poor women struggling to feed the children they already had. To patient after patient, the ob-gyn offered a solution: birth control. By patient after patient, she was asked to treat a different problem: "My husband's younger wife is pregnant, and I need a test to figure out why I am not getting pregnant too." The First-Worlder wanted to limit family size; the patients wanted fertility improve-ment. The ob-gyn told Glenn she could not in good conscience provide that, and went home frustrated.

If he could have, Glenn might have introduced the young ob-gyn to an elderly woman he had met in a clinic in Nigeria, who gently but pointedly raised the same issue. "For all of my lifetime, we know we have suffered from a problem called malaria," Glenn recalls the woman telling him. "But it was only when you white people came here that we heard we are suffering from a problem you call 'family.'" She wondered aloud why aid agencies sent fam-ily-planning literature to villages where malaria, not fertility, was the enemy.

"Health care is used by a lot of people as a coercive power, to get others to do what we want or think is best," Glenn later wrote in a journal entry. "On the missions I lead, we ask the people we're serving what *they* think would be in their best interests, and as much as possible, we help them attain those things, including when they conflict with our own interests. For me, it comes down to something pretty basic that is scriptural as well as philosophical. The Golden Rule is a pretty good standard. What kind of care do we provide? Well, what standard of care would I want for myself or my loved one?"

Glenn came to South Sudan in 2005, the same year that peace did—on paper.

From the time Sudan gained independence from Britain in 1956, Africa's largest nation had known only short seasons without conflict. In 1983, the military regime's attempt to impose Islamic Sharia law sparked a separatist rebellion in the south, home to the 30 percent of Sudanese who hold Christian or animist beliefs. Civil war raged for more than two decades. More than two million Sudanese died, and at least twice that many were displaced, including the storied Lost Boys of the Sudan, who walked hundreds of miles to reach refugee camps after their villages were destroyed.

In January 2005, with much fanfare, the Khartoum government and the Sudanese People's Liberation Movement signed the Comprehensive Peace Accord (CPA). It mandated a cease-fire, a power-sharing government, significant autonomy for the south, and future free elections. But when Glenn arrived in Sudan weeks later, and in the six missions he has made to the country since, conflict has been a constant. The peace accord reduced but did not eliminate skirmishes between rebel and government forces. Tens of thousands have died since 2003 in a separate war, decried worldwide as genocide, in the western region of Darfur.

And in South Sudan—a semi-autonomous region the size of France that has less than fifty miles of paved roads—villages were caught in both political crossfire and inter-tribal clashes that escalate from cattle raids to kidnappings and murders. In 2010, the first nationwide elections since the peace accord were widely decried as tainted, casting doubt on whether a 2011 referendum would go forward as scheduled to allow South Sudan residents to decide whether to become an independent nation.

Glenn has staged repeat missions to several villages in the region's northeastern provinces: Old Fangak, Duk Payuel, Werkok, Bor, Pibor. There, roots of tribal conflicts run deep into ancient cultures. Glenn studies the tribes' practices avidly and, when he can, proposes a medical or humanitarian solution to a culture-bred dilemma.

South Sudan's largest tribe is the Dinka people, some three million strong. The Nuer people, numbering two million, shared bloodlines with the Dinka centuries ago but now are rivals. And, in the areas where Glenn leads missions, both Dinka and Nuer are at war with a smaller clan, the 400,000-strong Murle. Though South Sudan sits atop massive oil preserves, its people are among the poorest on earth. Many are subsistence farmers, but the center of their existence—and their greatest joy—is their cattle.

In a Dinka creation myth Glenn finds especially telling, God gives the first Dinka man a choice. God will give the man cattle, whose virtues and value are clear—companionship, food, monetary value—or God will give the man another, unrevealed gift, the What. Though the man asks "What is the What?" God will not disclose. And so the man chooses the cattle, according a sacred status that the animals retain today.

Though Glenn would never say something so harsh to his Sudanese hosts, in his journal he is blunt: "Those cattle are the most damnable beasts! The people worship them. I have seen the mosquito bed nets sent by U.S. aid agencies to ward off malaria, and inside each bed net is not an infant but a calf. The cattle graze the land to desertification and leave a veneer of feces everywhere. They are economic drones. They do not pull anything because to hook up a cart or plow would be to abuse this wonderful animal. Many people don't eat them except when a bull is sacrificed for a wedding or other special event; some don't even milk them. All they do is stand there and look at them—that's their wealth, their bank account walking down the road."

Among these tribes, cattle raiding is commonplace. Conducting raids to capture rivals' cattle, and even children, is a traditional way to prove bravery and raise wealth and social standing—more sons to tend the cattle, more daughters who will fetch a bovine bride price. But for at least one tribe, Glenn learned, the raids have an additional urgency.

"The Murle have a big problem," Glenn noted after one of his first trips to the

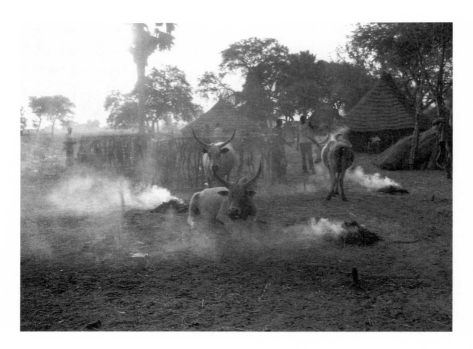

Though Glenn and mission colleagues aim always to respect local customs, in his journal Glenn criticizes the South Sudan cattle culture, in which the animals are "economic drones" that consume village resources and give little back.

region. "A very high rate of pelvic inflammatory disease, and that has given them infertility. If my older bride has PID and isn't fertile, I have to have a younger bride. So I have to steal other tribes' young girls and cattle—which amount to the same thing because with fifty cows, I can buy a bride. The Murle cattle raiders are the reason that every Nuer and Dinka who can get one has an AK-47."

To his Nuer and Dinka friends, Glenn suggested a plan. He would run a mission to the Murle, treat their PID and improve their fertility—and thus reduce their need to raid. The Nuer and Dinka were unconvinced: *No, you do not need to treat them; you need to kill them!*

Glenn declined, with a trademark phrase about his apolitical approach to medicine: "I can't tell a Murle from a Methodist at fifty paces. I just treat those in greatest need." He shelved the idea of the Murle mission, but he did not discard it.

During a mission to Malawi, Glenn picked up some of the brochures that world health groups had sent to promote HIV/AIDS education and prevention. It would be "a fascinating exercise," he later wrote, to help subsistence-living Malawians make sense of some of the brochures' statements about risk factors for HIV, including the following: "You cannot get AIDS from hot tubs."

Glenn considers such culturally ignorant health messages a shameful waste of resources, in countries where the virus has moved far faster than efforts to prevent it. But he takes heart from locals' homegrown efforts at HIV/AIDS education. When in Embangweni, his mission teams always attend at least one performance by a street-theater troupe that uses drama, song and dance to teach about prevention. He especially savors the name the troupe has taken, a time-honored expression in the native Timbuku language, *Tiko lera neko*. Translation: "We are all in this struggle together."

When Glenn was young, he had a gadget befitting a young scientist: an instrument that could separate spoken speech into its vowels and its consonants, creating two distinct streams of sound. Separating the sounds then was a parlor game. But since then, Glenn has learned the power of gestures, expressions and sounds—right down to vowels and consonants—to communicate across barriers of language and culture. He has written his own primer on "the communication I have all the time with patients, whether they are in the United States and we speak the same language or on another continent and we have no shared language.

If I give you the consonants, you might understand the subject matter, but you would have no idea how I felt about it. If I turn in the other direction and give you only the vowels, you might have no idea about the substance of something, but you'd know very much how I felt about it—you'd get that I was scolding you or soothing you or being emphatic with you. In Washington, D.C., a patient might not fully comprehend when I say I'm going to take out her adrenal gland, do this procedure with these specifics and these outcomes—the consonants. But she does understand that I'm holding her hand and telling her she'll be okay, the vowels. In Africa, I learn a few words of greeting in the local languages in every place I visit. Beyond that, folks may not understand one word I'm saying, but they get that I'm there to be helpful and reassuring, because I speak vowels.

A few years ago in the Philippines, I was to operate on a beautiful little nine-year-old girl who had a big lump under her chin. Her mother was really worried about her and knew only that I was about to put her to sleep and put her at risk. I went in and removed something in her thyroid gland that had developed separately from where it should have. Then I removed the breathing tube and picked her up to carry her, still sound asleep, to a recovery bed. I'm still wearing a gown and gloves with blood on them, so I don't have to re-scrub; Mama sees me carrying the limp body of her daughter and she is scared to death. But I bring her over and put her in bed, turn her head to the side so she won't aspirate. And I lean over and through my mask, I give her a kiss on the cheek. Mama loses it because then she understands not only that her daughter is okay, but that she is appreciated. She comes over and gives her daughter a kiss, and we hug. That's the end of our conversation right there.

The following morning, really early, I am not even out of bed and I'm told there is someone waiting outside. The girl still has *the dressing on and an IV in; she is pushing the IV trolley. I learn later that she and Mama have been rehearsing with one of the English-speaking nurses. She comes forward and stands on tiptoes. I lean down and she says to me, 'Happy Valentine's Day!' And she throws her arms around my neck and gives me a kiss.*

Recognize what has happened here. I talked vowels to Mama. Mama got that, no translation needed. She went back, found someone who could teach these three English words, and brought her daughter, before it even was dawn, to recite this line. She has come two-thirds of the way in my direction; she has learned that this day is an occasion in my culture, learned words in my language and embraced me. I had a profound communication with Mama and this child, neither of whom spoke my language — but they got my vowels, and the consonants they learned were for the sake of speaking back to me. That moment with that little girl pretty much summarizes what I was there for.

Even the most skeptical citizens of Assa and the neighboring villages could see the results of the Goiter Project, especially with the young whose lack of iodine had caused the mental and physical stunting known as cretinism. Diane Downing vividly recalls how "before the iodine treatments, the cretins would just sit on a log all day; as dear as they were, their families were totally waiting on them for everything in life. But with the iodine, many would be able to carry a little wood or water, or hoe in the garden."

As the treatments were administered in more and more villages—Ebali, Banda, Ndamana—Glenn relished not just the health gains but also the educational opportunities. Giving villagers the iodine that their foods lacked

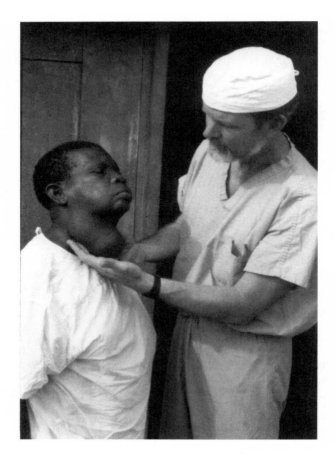

Though Glenn and other volunteers made some headway teaching Assa's villagers what caused their goiters and cretinism—the "what" of hypothyroidism—they never completely dispelled villagers' beliefs that the "why" of the disease involves curses, divine retribution and other non-medical causes.

opened the way to teach about nutrition. Showing patients how their goiters could be reduced led to broader conversations about wellness.

But for all that Glenn could teach the Congolese about combating disease, he could not shake their culturally ingrained beliefs about what caused it. Or so he concluded, in an essay he titled "The Lion, the Pastor and the Cretin: A Study in Causation of Disease":

A lion? Right in the middle of Ndamana village, dragging a man out of his hut at night? This story would bear looking into.

The pastor and his wife lived in a dominant hut in the center of Ndamana village. When an assistant pastor was assigned from outside the village, there was some confrontation over roles and limits of authority. But in this small community — hardly more than a wide spot in the trail leading toward the border with the Central African Republic (CAR) — the pastor and his wife remained prominent citizens.

There is not much "evening" in this equatorial location. After the single meal of the day at dusk, the fires sputter out and it is time to retire into the shelter of the thatched hut. This the pastor and his wife did and soon were fast asleep, lying quite close together on a wickerwork bed.

It was some time at night when the wife woke up, screaming with pain. Something had seized her foot, and she would not have awakened for the inconvenience of insect stings, nor even rat or snake bite. Her screams woke up her husband, who sat bolt upright and seemed to understand in an instant what was happening. He uttered one exclamation — "Praise God!!" — before his skull was crushed in the darkness, quite audibly next to the ears of his terrified wife.

The big male lion had first attacked the wife but then, when her husband stirred, had closed its powerful jaws over the pastor's head. The wife saw the beast give her husband's limp body a shake then begin dragging it from the hut.

Villagers roused by the wife's screams peered out of their huts to see in the moonlight a dark shadow dragging a body by the head, carelessly stepping on the dangling limbs until it left the clearing and disappeared into the bush. There were sounds of thrashing and dragging as the lion retreated farther from Ndamana, then the even more frightening sounds of dismemberment and bone crunching as the lion fed. The wife continued to scream and ululate, her cries mingling with her neighbors' wails of mourning.

Some men emerged from their huts and stirred the dying embers to make fire brands and torches, not to follow the lion's trail but to attempt to ward off his return. No one slept in Ndamana for the rest of the night, each villager cowering in his or her own thoughts. In a neighboring hut, some of the women attended to the pastor's wife, binding up the bleeding stump where the lion had bitten off most of her foot.

When dawn arrived, a band of village men gingerly advanced down the wide, bloody drag line into the bush. They had gone only three hundred meters when they found the pastor's half-eaten corpse, without evidence of the lion's presence at that moment. They pulled the remains from the bush and hurried back to the village, where their arrival renewed the mourners' wailing. The widow was spared the sight of what was left of her husband, having been taken to the river crossing for emergency care, and then transferred to a clinic in the CAR.

With all haste lest the lion return and as much formality as could be mustered by the assistant pastor, a grave was dug. The

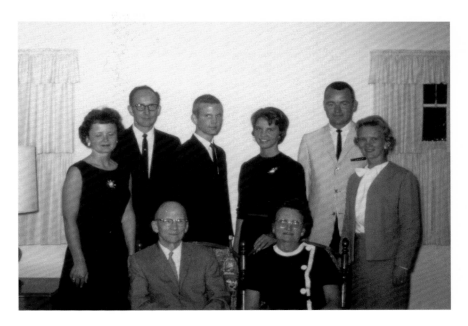

A 1964 portrait of Bill and Alice Geelhoed (seated) and family: from left, Martheen and Don Griffioen, Glenn Geelhoed, Milly Geelhoed, Arnie and Shirley Snoeyink.

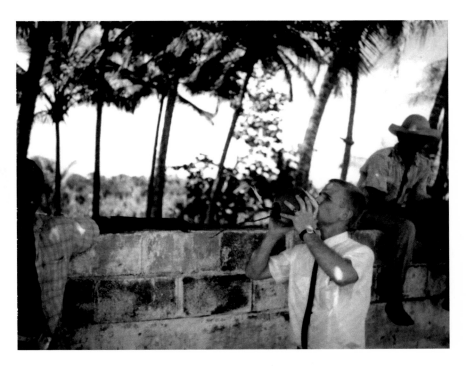

Glenn samples coconut milk on his first foreign medical mission trip to the Dominican Republic.

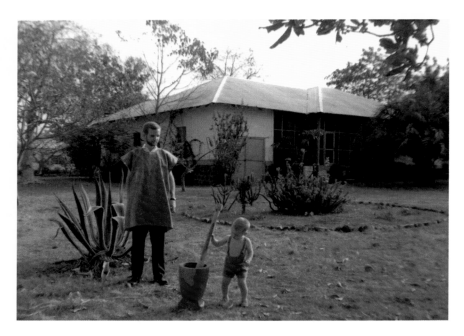

On the grounds of Nigeria's Takum Christian Hospital, Glenn (in a traditional Nigerian tunic) plays with Donald, who turned two during the 1968 mission trip.

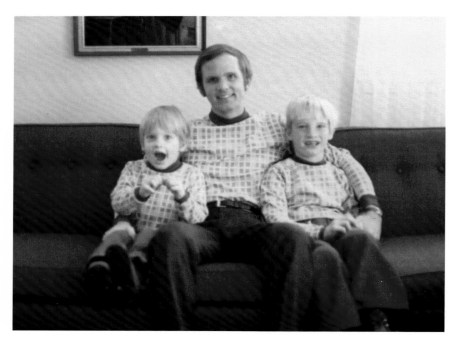

Michael, Glenn and Donald Geelhoed in 1974, in matching shirts Glenn's mother made.

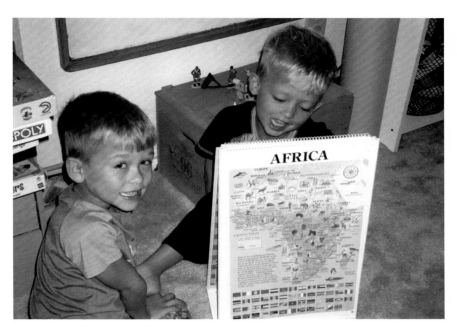

Glenn's twin grandsons Jordan (left) and Devin use maps to track their grandfather's African mission travels.

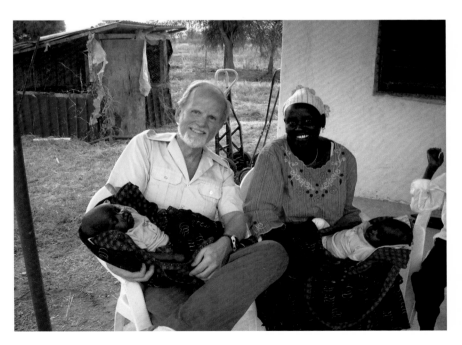

Glenn poses with a midwife and her twin sons in Werkok, Sudan, January 2009.

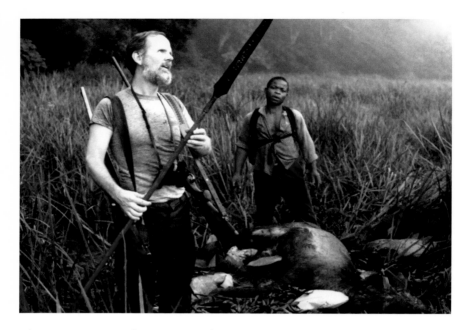

Glenn examines a spear his Assa, Congo, hunting companions use.

Glenn returned from Africa during his 1996 Fulbright Year to run the historic 100th Boston Marathon.

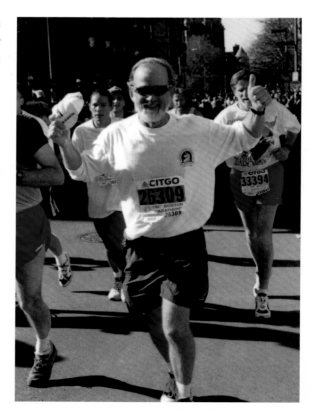

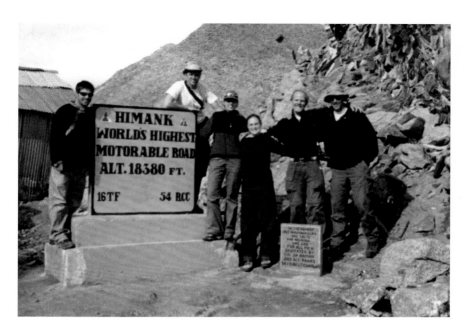

Glenn and mission colleagues in Ladakh, northern India, at a Himalayan landmark where climbers leave colorful prayer flags.

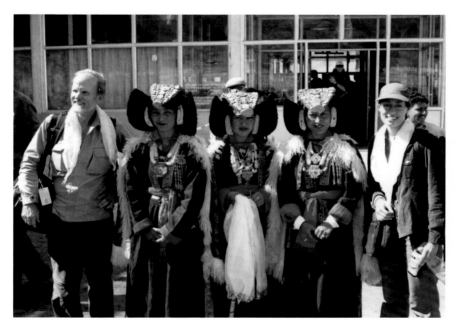

Glenn and mission participant Elizabeth Yellen (in cap) flank Ladakhi women in traditional garb at a reception for the Tangste Clinic.

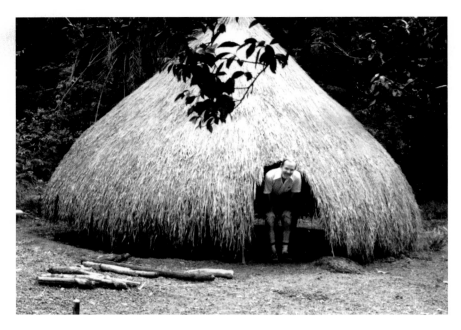

Glenn emerges from the hut in Ndamana, Congo, where a lion attacked a couple, injuring the wife and killing the husband, the village pastor.

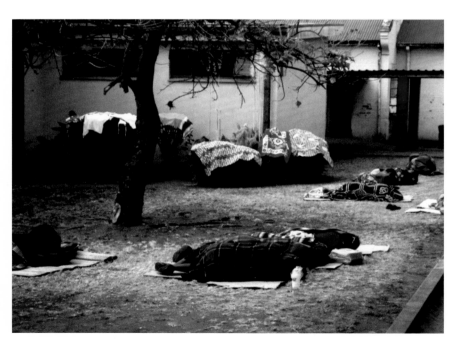

When Swaziland's Raleigh Fitkin Memorial Hospital reached capacity during Glenn's missions there, patients were housed in the open-air courtyard.

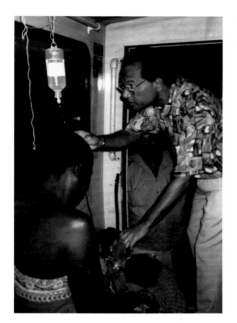
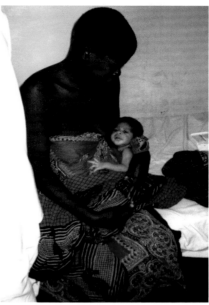

In Mozambique, Glenn photographed a mercy mission: the "good Mama" and baby that he and colleague Dr. Ivo Garrido (in patterned shirt) took by train to a hospital for emergency surgery.

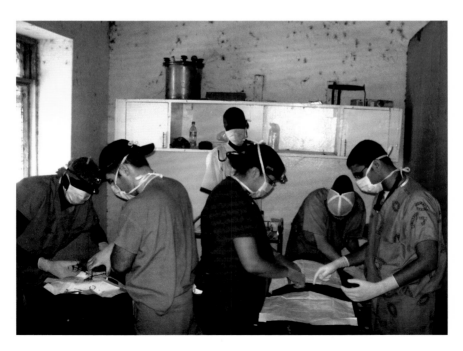

Glenn's mission team members and local practitioners work together in an Old Fangak, Sudan, operating room.

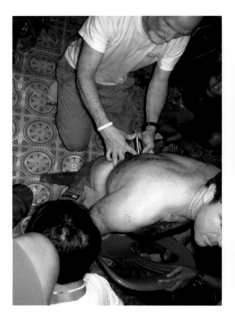
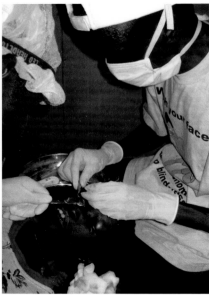

Glenn's missions emphasize locals and visitors teaching each other. **Above left:** *He demonstrates a lumbar puncture on a mission team member in Burma.* **Above right:** *A Sudanese practitioner shows others how to perform a blindness-prevention procedure Glenn taught him.*

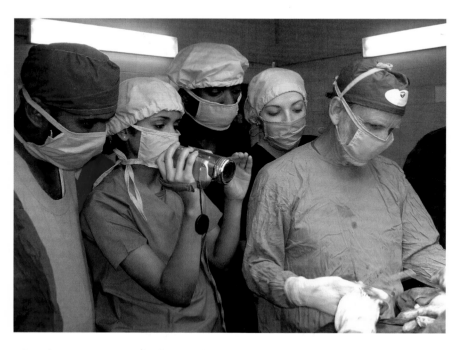

Glenn demonstrates surgical technique while students observe on a 2009 mission to Khartoum Teaching Hospital in Sudan.

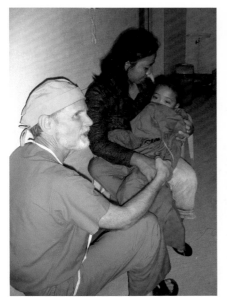
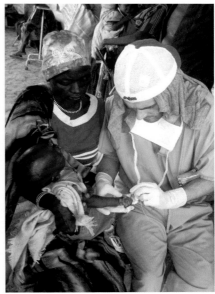

Above left: In the Far North Luzon General Hospital and Training Center in the Philippines in 2009, Glenn comforts a mother whose child has pneumonia. Above right: Medical student Will Schmitt tends a patient at an open-air wound clinic in Old Fangak, Sudan, in 2009.

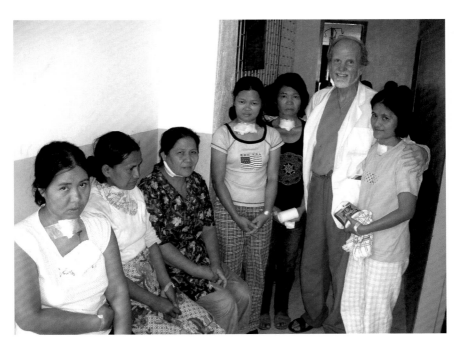

Patients whose goiters he has removed pose with Glenn in the Tiboli clinic in Mindanao, during a 2008 mission to the Philippines.

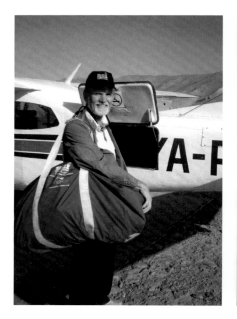

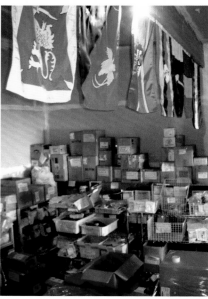

Above left: Glenn beside the chartered Cessna that carried mission personnel and duffels of supplies to remote Lal, Afghanistan. Above right: In the Project S.A.V.E. warehouse, donated medical supplies await shipment to needy developing-world health care operations.

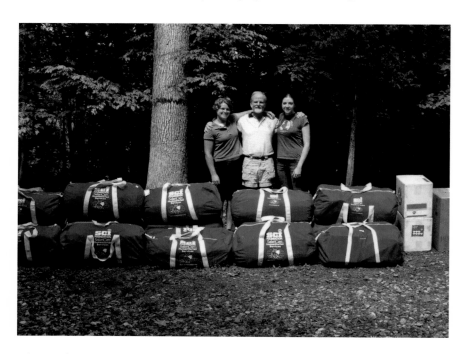

Glenn and 2007 mission participants Johanna Hasler (left) and Julie Whitis, with bags of supplies bound for Ethiopia, Sudan and Chad.

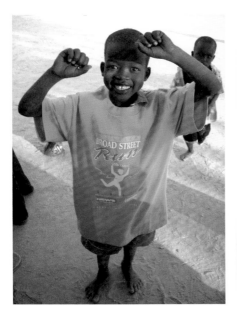 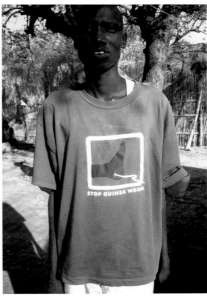

Above left: *A boy in Werkok, Sudan, with probably the first new piece of clothing he ever received: one of the race T-shirts Glenn and fellow runner Imme Dyson save to distribute during missions.*
Above right: *The T-shirt of a health aide in Old Fangak, Sudan, promotes the eradication of guinea worm, cause of one of the many parasitic diseases that plague the world's "bottom billion."*

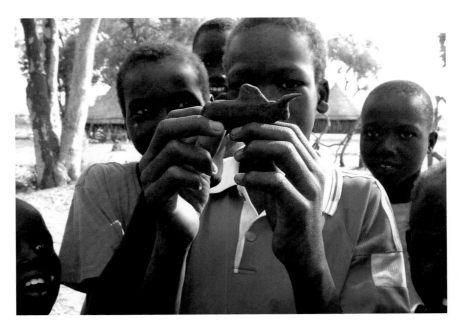

In cattle cultures of South Sudan, as they have for centuries, boys tend their families' herds and use clay cows as playthings.

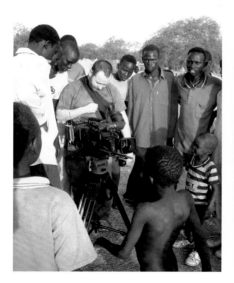
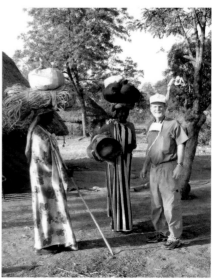

Above left: Old Fangak, Sudan, villagers line up to peer through the camera lens of the documentary film crew that accompanied Glenn's December 2009–January 2010 mission. *Above right:* Glenn greets women carrying their handicrafts to market in Old Fangak.

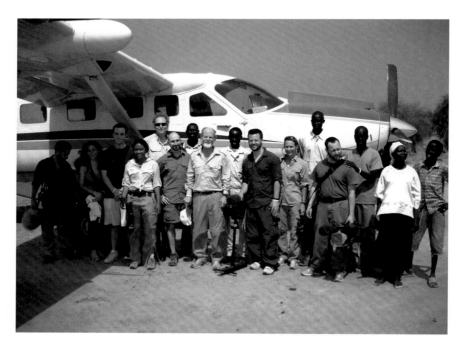

Members of Glenn's December 2009–January 2010 mission that included a documentary film crew and "medical diplomacy" overtures to warring Dinka and Murle tribal leaders.

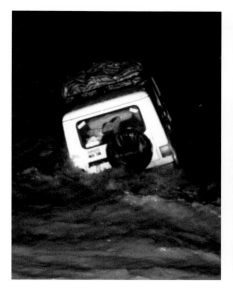
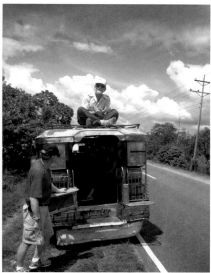

Vehicles figure in many of Glenn's mission adventures. **Above left:** *The jeep that got stuck in a creek in the Himalayas and had to be pushed out by Glenn and other mission members.* **Above right:** *Glenn waits atop an overheated jeepney on the way to a mission stop in Mindanao, the Philippines.*

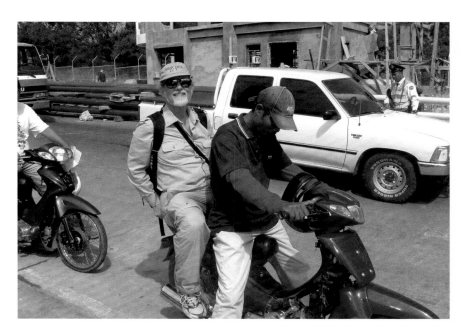

Glenn acquires "local transport" in January 2008 to see the sights in southern Mindanao, the Philippines.

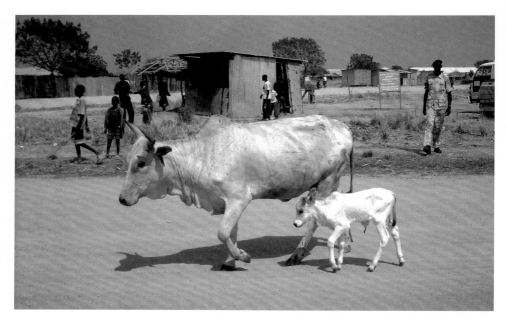

Glenn admits frustration with aspects of South Sudan's cattle culture, in which the animals are revered and pampered while their owners endure hunger and hardship.

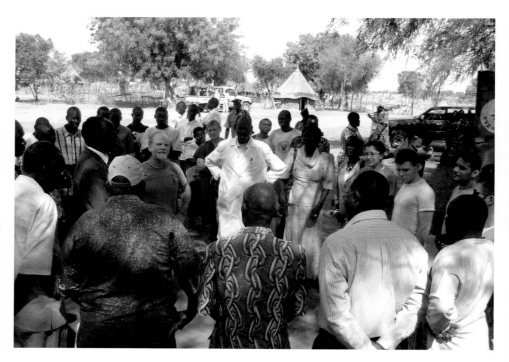

Glenn meets with chiefs and the commissioner of Duk Payuel, Sudan, to receive thanks for past medical missions and requests for future ones.

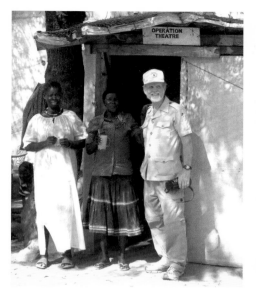
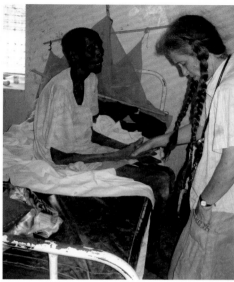

Above left: *Glenn and residents of Bor, Sudan, pose under the "operating theater" sign of a bombed-out former hospital building that medical mission organizations hope to help locals restore.* *Above right:* *In Old Fangak, Sudan, Dr. Jill Seaman checks on a tuberculosis patient during a visit by one of Glenn's mission teams.*

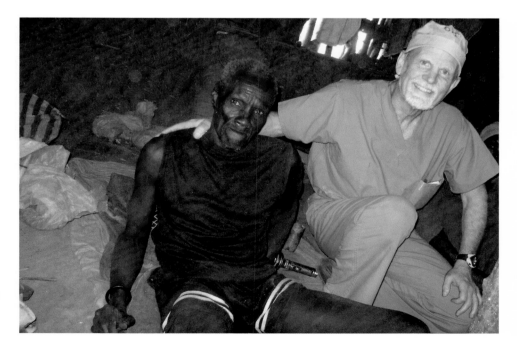

Glenn makes what he terms "a hut call" on the Old Fangak, Sudan, village blacksmith, recovering from paralysis after treatment for tuberculosis of the spine.

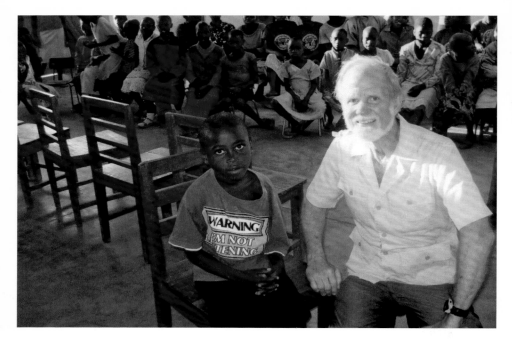

"Warning: I'm Not Listening": Glenn appreciated the joke on a boy's T-shirt at a school for the deaf he visits during missions to Embangweni, Malawi.

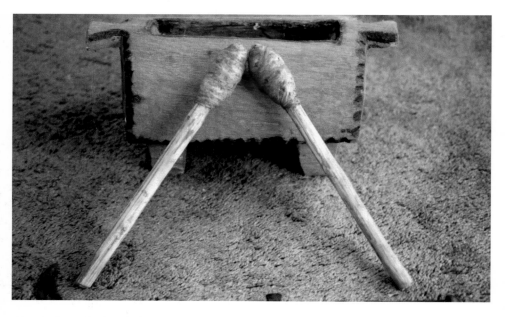

Glenn's photo of a cherished gift from his visits to Assa, Congo: A miniature "talking drum" that master drummer Bule carved for him.

pastor's remains were interred not far from the hut in which he had lain down to sleep for the last time.

The assistant pastor dispatched a runner to the district office, which sent reinforcements to assist the village men. That night, as the men lay in wait at the site where the pastor's remains were found, the lion returned. In an instant, the big beast was riddled with spears. Snarling and roaring, he retreated into the brush, where he soon was heard gurgling and gasping, and then nothing. A brave villager approached to verify the kill, touching a spear to the lion's eye until it no longer blinked. He was a very large, black-maned male lion, with very worn-down incisors but no other signs of what his history may have been before he turned man-eater.

Triumphant and relieved but still numb at the pastor's loss, the men dragged the lion back to the village. Women filed out to see the dead beast and curse and spit upon it. Young men not present at the kill took turns spearing the dead body until there was little of the perforated hide to be saved.

In the local language, the word widow means literally "poor person." Women are not allowed to own anything, and the dead man's properties are divided among his male siblings. The typical fate for a widow the age of the pastor's wife is a very short and unhappy life, even more so if she is crippled.

With the aid of a stick, the pastor's widow began learning to hobble on the stump of what had been her foot. But suffering depression from the loss of her husband and her social status, she had very little will to live. Within a few weeks after the event, the village women knew nothing of her whereabouts.

Though the pastor's hut was prime real estate in the center of Ndamana, there was some talk of burning it. Others suggested performing a purification rite to dispel the evil that befell its inhabitants. Only when I inquired further did I understand the village dynamics that surrounded the fatal hut, the lion, the pastor — and one more.

In the week preceding the fateful night, during the course of a worship service, the pastor had let fly at the assistant pastor a threat, to keep him in his place. Rather than responding directly to this challenge, the assistant pastor began an impassioned litany bewailing his own misfortune. After a prolonged period of infertility and stillbirths, his wife had conceived and delivered a son, a source of great joy upon his arrival. However, it was becoming increasingly apparent that the child was a full-blown cretin, developmentally retarded in mental, social and physical milestones, and would not be a contributing member of the family that his father had so desperately longed for.

The assistant pastor did not speak of a condition. Rather, he thundered about a curse. He knew who had visited this curse upon him, he said (and all knew who he meant). And he closed with a prophecy that a sure sign from God would befall the evildoer who had robbed him of his healthy child.

The Goiter Project team had worked for years to illuminate the causes of a major medical problem. But all our efforts became minimally interesting and massively irrelevant the moment the black-maned lion entered the pastor's hut. Centuries-old beliefs about cause, effect and retribution were underscored beyond contradiction by a signal event so obvious and self-evident that no explanation was needed and no refutation was possible.

We could tell the people of Ndamana anything we wished about the "what" of cretinism. But as to its "why," for what more proof could one ask?

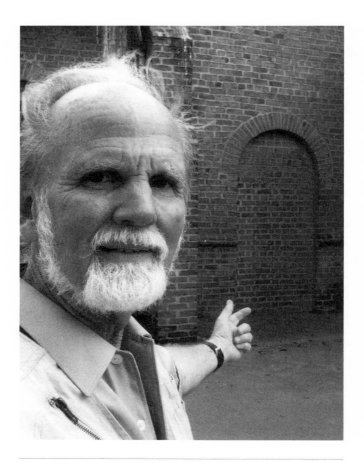

On his exercise runs during missions in Malawi, Glenn became curious about a bricked-up side door in a local church. When he inquired, he learned the door had been added so lepers would not mingle with other congregants, and later bricked up—but not for the reason he might have hoped.

CHAPTER TWELVE

Bricking Up the Leper Door

GLENN LAUNCHES EVERY MISSION WITH THE SAME REMINDER TO participants: Indigenous peoples' cultures, beliefs and customs must be treated with respect. And yet, on some missions, Glenn and colleagues run up against culturally ordained practices and attitudes that they find hard to countenance. In these cases, team members walk a tricky line: How to behave with integrity when their host culture's ways are repugnant; how to respond, as healers, to customs they deem destructive.

Glenn knows he and team members can't always invoke "doctor's orders" against cultural norms, even those that are lethally ignorant or cruel. "But sometimes," he tells them, "we are morally bound to try. And sometimes, we prevail."

His repeat visits to remote reaches of the Congo placed Glenn in the footsteps of another adventurous Midwesterner. Earl Dix, a self-described farm boy from Butte, Nebraska, was twenty-five when he felt "God's leading" to become a missionary. In 1929, with his fiancée, Helena, his "varmint rifle" and a few other worldly goods, Dix sailed to Africa.

The couple established a mission outpost on a hill in the village of Banda, building first a church, then a school and then a hospital. During more than a half century of service, Dix (who died in 1983) became "Papa Dix" to his flock. He tended not only to their spiritual needs but their physical ones with meat from the big game he hunted.

Learning that the root of the local Rauwolfia plant was the source of a drug used to treat high blood pressure, Dix sent locals into the bush to gather it. Then he sold it to European pharmaceutical companies. With the proceeds, Dix paid for mission projects including students' schooling. He even sent a few young men away for specialized medical training. And so it was that one of Papa's former students became one of Glenn's chief assistants during Congo medical missions.

His family named him Ngbamboligbe Kunangbangate; in the local Pazande dialect, it means "God is so much good, but man is bad." Choosing a less daunting name as he grew, the young man called himself Andre; and after training in bush dentistry and mouth, head and neck specialties, he was widely known as Andre the Dentiste.

When Andre accompanied Glenn to Banda in 1996, it was his first trip home in more than a decade. For the occasion, Andre wore his only coat and tie. Peddling a bicycle with one tire-less wheel, Andre's younger brother arrived bearing their elderly father. The elder had had part of his foot amputated to remove an "African melanoma"—a cancer that occurs in less pigmented areas of black skin such as under toenails. But still the cancer had advanced. Before the visit, Glenn had obtained a precious few tablets of a chemotherapy drug called cyclophosphamide. "Not very good against this cancer," he wrote in a journal entry, "but it was all that we had. So we brought it and gave it to Andre's father."

The next day, Glenn, Andre and his father were at the hospital when a woman carried in her young daughter. The child had an obvious, advanced case of Burkitt's Lymphoma, a jaw tumor that causes enormous swelling of the lower face. Glenn explained that while the condition looked horrendous, this particular cancer actually was exquisitely sensitive to chemotherapy of even the simplest sort. As little as a single dose of the

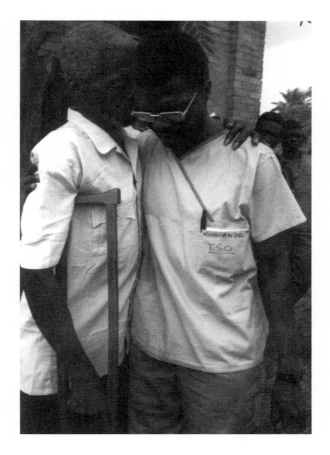

On a 1996 medical mission, one of Glenn's assistants was a young Congolese medical and dental trainee, Andre, who was visiting his home village after years away at school. Glenn snapped a photo of Andre embracing his father, who was dying of a cancer for which Glenn and Andre had brought medicine they hoped might slow the disease, but that they knew could not cure it.

cyclophosphamide, he noted, had been known to make the tumor fade away, sometimes nearly overnight.

Andre and his father went away a little distance for a consultation. Speaking in Pazande with their arms around each other, they made a touching picture, the proud father embracing his accomplished son. When Andre returned to Glenn, he repeated the conversation. "Did the American professor say that this drug I have might save that little girl's life?" his father had

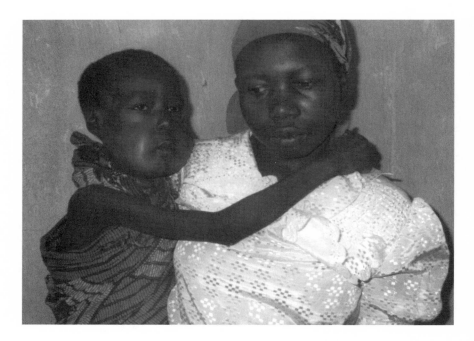

A Congolese mother holds her daughter, whose face is disfigured by Burkitt's Lymphoma. When Glenn and local health worker Andre brought a medication that was likelier to be effective for the girl than for Andre's father's cancer, the father insisted on donating it rather than taking it himself. But first, village elders had to rule on whether the girl should get the treatment.

asked. Then he handed the tablets back to Andre, saying "It is all for the best!"

"Who else would be this heroic under the same circumstances?" Glenn wrote of the moment. "They were passing this chance for life along, from one who had the pills in his possession but had had a long and good life and did not have much hope extending from them, to another who had only got eight years into life but would not go eight days more without some kind of miraculous treatment."

Glenn told the mother that this drug could save her daughter's life and should be administered as soon as possible. The mother said she understood, took the packet of pills and left. When Glenn asked Andre what would happen next, he was told the facts of life in this community: The mother is "only a woman," and women in this culture do not make decisions as important as whether this medicine might be taken, even when the decision concerns whether their own child lives or dies. Such decisions must be brought up before the elder males, who will decide whether she takes the treatment or not.

Fair enough, Glenn thought. *Go with what you know, but be quick about it.* Before he left to go on to Assa, Glenn's parting words to Andre were, "There is not a lot of time for deliberation, for without the medicine her life will surely be short."

A few months passed and when Glenn asked after the child, Andre reported she had died. The doctor pressed for details: Was the treatment given too late? The protégé, eyes cast down, explained that the treatment was not given. The Azande elders had made their plans: First, they would do a divination ceremony to learn who or what had caused the child to be ill; then they would deliberate as to whether the child should be given this Western medicine or some other treatment. While they were scheduling the ceremony, the child died.

Glenn's notes in his journal were edged with bitterness: "Notwithstanding the wonderful coincidence of visitors from another planet dropping in with this lifesaving medicine, she was an Azande girl, so this would have to be resolved the Azande way." And so it was. Against all his work to spread understanding of what caused and cured disease, Glenn scored this as a loss: *Africa one, modern medicine zero.*

—

Landlocked and largely desert, the impoverished nation of Chad has been called "the dead heart of Africa." Since gaining independence from France in 1960, it has endured invasions by its neighbor to the north, Libya; a flood of refugees from Darfur, across its eastern border with Sudan; three decades of civil war; numerous contested elections; and fitful periods of peace broken by rebel campaigns. When Glenn led a medical mission to Chad in summer 2007, a nationwide strike had closed all government medical facilities for six weeks and counting.

Greeting Glenn's team at the airport was Scott Downing—the son of

Glenn's Goiter Project colleague, Diane Downing—who as a teen had assisted Glenn during operations in Assa. Scott Downing had settled his young family in majority-Muslim Chad to work with the Evangelical Church of Chad in the southeastern town of Am Timan.

With Downing providing introductions, Glenn's team sought government permission to open just one hospital in Am Timan for just eight days, so the visitors could provide surgical care for a waiting list of patients. The government allowed the hospital to open; it warned hospital employees they would not be paid extra to assist Glenn's team, but employees showed up anyway, to work and learn. And so began what Glenn called "the Miracle Mission," long days in the operating room addressing long-neglected conditions and medical emergencies.

Glenn's approach to working in Chad made an impression on all who met him, says Downing. "It goes against the culture here for someone with his authority to be willing to walk the town, or bounce around in the back of an open pickup truck; to sit on the floor writing in his journal, or to roll up his sleeves and help clean the OR after a particularly messy operation. Most here take advantage of their position of relative authority to sit back and be served. But Glenn comes to serve. That was apparent to all. His genuine desire to help people get better was obvious, and his willingness to tackle the difficult cases in less-than-ideal conditions was contagious."

As Downing assisted Glenn's team, he also was struck by how "Glenn is always looking for ways to develop people's capacity. He would select someone in the operating block to teach them a specific surgical procedure. He was putting the scalpel in their newly trained hands for future days when he would not be available. That's what brings him joy and drives him."

The Chad trip was the fourth medical mission in eighteen months for Julie Whitis. At GWU, Texas-born Whitis had completed her international-affairs degree and taken a research job, but she hadn't entirely relinquished "the dream of medical school. I wanted to be like a Doctors Without Borders person. And then I met Glenn, who seemed to be kind of his own doctor without borders." Whitis worked with Glenn on medical missions in 2006 to Rwanda and Eritrea, and in 2007 to Sudan and Chad.

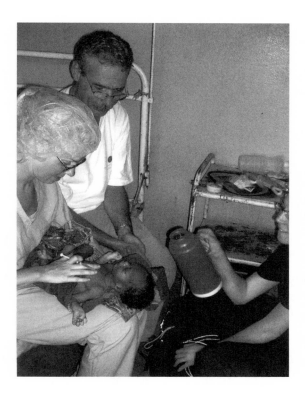

Am Timan, Chad, 2007: Mission team members Sarah Brown, Tim Harrison and Julie Whitis with "Baby Tim," the infant who would have died without the team's insistent efforts to feed and rehydrate him.

In Am Timan, "We hadn't been at the hospital for more than an hour," Whitis recalls, "when this woman arrived. She had been in labor for what sounded like days and she needed an emergency C-section. When her baby came out, he was just purple, no signs of life.

"We managed to revive the child, but he was so worn out from the lengthy birth process. And the father—it was the male relatives making the decisions—kept just putting the baby down and not attending to him saying, *'Insha'Allah, Insha'Allah'*—'if it's God's will.' They basically threw up their arms and shrugged their shoulders.

"That was really hard for me to take. I knew the biology of what was going on. I knew why this baby was not strong. We said to the family, 'If you just feed him a little bit, he'll pick up, but he'll never gain his strength if you don't work with him.' And they just said, *'Insha'Allah.'*

"We tried very much to respect their culture. But in that case we all kind of voted to be the pushy Americans and play dumb: 'Sorry, we don't know what your words mean. We're going to come in and check on the baby, and while we're here, we're going to feed him a little bit.' They kept wrapping him up in all these blankets—in the Sahara—and the poor baby is sweating and probably getting dehydrated. We mixed up a rehydration solution and fed him every time we went by, with a syringe. We went by every hour and didn't take the translators with us, we just kind of barged in.

"Long story short, the child ended up making it. After the required period of waiting to be sure that he survived, they named the baby Tim, after one of the nurses on our mission team. But the whole attitude toward babies was really difficult for me to take, as was the treatment of women."

The treatment of women. To Glenn, a lover of irony and wordplay, the phrase is ripe with meanings. He enters cultures where the norm is second-class treatment of women. Then, wherever possible, he overrides the norm to insure excellent medical treatment of women.

In Afghanistan, many Middle Eastern countries, and in heavily Muslim African countries such as Ethiopia, Somaliland, Sudan and Chad, by religious law Glenn should not speak to women let alone operate on them. And yet he finds ways. In journal notes, his glee at pulling this off is evident: "Almost all my interactions with women in these countries violate cultural norms—but I'm forgiven because I do it with therapeutic intent."

On missions, one of the most common operations Glenn performs is exclusively on women: the repair of vesicovaginal fistula, or VVF. Though the injury is rare in developed countries with modern obstetric care, the World Health Organization reports high prevalence of VVF throughout the developing world—in virtually all of Africa and south Asia as well as parts of Oceana, Latin America, the Middle East and Central Asia.

Women who are young, undernourished or both, whose pelvises have not reached full growth, may be unable to deliver a baby vaginally after days or even weeks of trying. During the prolonged, obstructed labor, tissue begins to die and tear, leaving an opening, or fistula, between the urinary bladder and the vagina. The VVF permits a constant, uncontrolled leaking of urine into the vagina that turns women into the lepers of modernity: soiled, smelly pariahs, typically disowned by their husbands and cast out of their homes.

Glenn's most memorable patient in Chad was a beautiful fourteen-year-old girl—*too small and young to be pregnant*, he thought as soon as he saw her. By the time she was brought to the operating room, she had labored for two weeks, the baby was long dead, and a quarter-sized hole had opened between her bladder and vagina.

"The girl is lying on the table, prepped for the repair operation," Glenn wrote in his journal. "I ask the interpreter to explain to her that when I inject the spinal anesthesia through a lumbar puncture, it is going to hurt, and I squeeze her hand. She stares off into space with a look that says, 'What do you think you could possibly do that would hurt me?' The most world-weary woman I had ever seen. She has had no relationship to men except for exploitation—first her father who sold her into marriage and then the husband who thought she'd be good for a few children. But she couldn't drive a baby through that tiny, child-sized pelvis, so the husband complains to the father, 'You sold me bad goods!' and throws her out. Now here she is in the stirrups, there's another male touching her, and she's got two or three other people looking at her. But the difference is, every one of us is here in her best interest."

Even by Glenn's standards, the operation is a complicated one: carefully stretching and stitching torn flesh, insuring blood supply to the repair site, placing tissue grafts. Every step is described as it is performed, to his team members who might never see this procedure again and to the locals who need to learn to perform it. With the repairs successfully completed and the girl moved to a recovery room, Glenn gathers staff for post-op care instructions, chief among them that no one is to release the girl until he clears it.

A man approaches Glenn—the patient's father, Glenn is told. Translators are summoned; the girl's female relatives stand within earshot, veiled, silent. The father says he must take his daughter home the next day. Glenn explains her healing will take several days in the hospital and several more weeks at home. The father insists: He must take her because tomorrow she

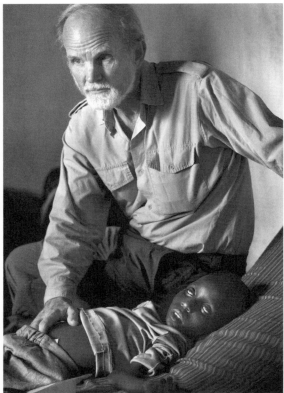

Photo: Stephen M. Katz/PHP

Glenn checks on a gravely ill child during a 2006 mission to Rwanda. A colleague from the Rwanda mission, Julie Whitis, says what team members witness during missions leaves them "changed forever. It kills you a little bit—but it also motivates you."

is to marry a new husband, who already has paid the bride price. No, says Glenn, not possible.

The father presses: If not tomorrow, then when *can* she be married? Glenn's first, angry response—grasped even before it is translated—is "Never, you bastard!" He knows he cannot enforce that, but his vehemence buys time and emboldens the girls' female relatives. He repeats his instructions to them: the post-op care, the recuperation period. They understand, the translator says, and they will do their best to see to it. The father leaves, irate. A week later, when Glenn's mission is ending, the girl is ready to go home, continent and healing well. Her fate beyond that, Glenn knew, would depend on which proved stronger: the protectiveness of her female relatives or the profit motivation of her father.

From the Chad mission, Julie Whitis remembers the VVF patient, baby Tim and numerous other cases that outraged her, as a woman and a health professional. "In other countries, there would have been some kind of child protective services, someone to speak on their behalf, but there was nothing," she says. From the Rwanda mission, she remembers "the twelve-year-old children walking around without arms, and you know someone maimed them when they were babies. There's no other way to describe it—it's just pure, cold evil. If you're a person of goodwill, you can't see things like that and not be changed forever. It kills you a little bit.

"But it also motivates you," she went on, "in different ways for different people. It was so amazing to see how we could touch the lives of people, especially with surgery where you can go in and fix somebody on the spot. That's awesome, and I understand how Glenn will never want to give that up. But for myself, it's not where I think I can make the most impact.

"For me, what I saw motivated me to come back and try to participate in fixing these things from the top down. We need both types of people—the people out there in the field fixing the VVFs, but also the people working at the community level and the ministerial level, on policy change and social change."

Whitis enrolled in an accelerated Johns Hopkins University program, earning a two-year master's degree in public health in just eleven months. After graduation, she joined the air force, to work as a public-health officer on postings with her fiancé, a medical student and air force officer. She is determined to continue working on international health issues. Since the medical missions, Whitis says, "it doesn't feel like a choice any more—more like a calling. Once you have experienced this, you have to do something."

Glenn likes to say he is anthropologist enough not to obsess over cultural differences, with one notable exception. "I do not object to tribal markings, or a bone through the nose or a lip plate," he once wrote. "But I have never understood how any civilization can throw away or waste the better parts of half its population"—the half that is female.

The eighteen-year-old woman arrived at Embangweni Hospital with a severe bowel obstruction. With her was her nine-week-old daughter, hungry and crying to nurse. Though Glenn and Elizabeth Yellen rushed the mother to the operating room, the entire bowel was black from lack of blood flow, and the woman could not be saved. So Glenn turned next to the daughter—still hungry, still crying, now motherless—and looked for a way to feed her.

Glenn proposed finding another woman who would suckle the orphaned girl. But while wet-nursing was common in some countries, it was not the custom in Embangweni; another solution would have to be found.

A sign on the Embangweni Hospital door lintel, declaring the facility "a baby-friendly hospital," showed a baby bottle slashed with the international symbol for "No." Glenn understood why global aid agencies promoted breast feeding unstintingly in nations where formula was over-marketed, largely unnecessary and costly, and the water to mix it with often unsafe. But he also understood that the principled, well-reasoned policy meant nothing right now to the hungry baby, nor to other nursing children whose mothers left Embangweni on the cemetery oxcarts.

In the hospital break room, Glenn tried to make a little "milk" with coffee whitener to tide the child over, but nowhere in the hospital could he find a bottle or rubber nipple. He finally took a driver and ambulance into town, came back with some baby formula, and recruited the dead woman's sister into an elaborate charade. When Auntie appeared to be modestly covering her chest with a draped cloth as the baby nursed, she actually was covering a bottle of formula suspended between her breasts. Had the bottle-feeding been discovered, the hospital could have lost its "baby-friendly" certification and aid funding. But as far as Glenn knew, the work-around never was discovered, and was repeated occasionally as necessary.

Glenn recorded the moral of the story in his journal:

The untoward consequence of "doing good" when you're uninformed
is that it bites you in the backside every time. By uninformed, I mean

not understanding the circumstances: The people who sat at a board-room table and said, "Baby-friendly means never bottle-feeding" did not understand that in Embangweni, that policy might scratch a hundred nursing children whose mothers had died. Their goal was to set down principles. When we gave that child a bottle — as a "crime," under wraps — our goal was to take care of a human being.

The U.S. President's Emergency Plan for AIDS Relief (PEPFAR) program has spent tens of billions of dollars since 2003 on HIV/AIDS prevention and treatment. But even where there is greater understanding of the virus, there often is no less stigma. In many of the hardest-hit African nations, AIDS is considered so shameful that people refuse to be tested even if they believe they've been exposed. And those who confirm they are HIV-positive often keep their status secret, lest employers, neighbors and relatives shun or persecute them.

Traveling throughout Africa in recent decades, Glenn has witnessed AIDS sweeping the continent. He has watched how Africans watch each other for signs of the dread disease; he has learned the veiled references, the euphemisms used to avoid calling it by name. "He's got a puncture," for example, means a man went from plump to skeletal as quickly as if a pinprick had let the air out of him, from the wasting of late-stage AIDS.

Glenn's work in Malawi placed him at the intersection of the present-day plague of AIDS and another plague that preceded it: leprosy. He reflected on that in an essay:

I noticed it on the run. As dawn was breaking over the Malawi savannah, I was returning from an early morning run along the bush roads around Loudon Station. The station church was the first structure built in this area, designed, planned and overseen by Robert Loudon, friend and compatriot of the Scottish missionary and explorer David Livingstone. The very large edifice, bigger than anything within a radius of several hundred kilometers, was capped by a spire atop a steeple on the roof. Construction was completed in 1902 with a few modifications to the original design, one of them particularly poignant: an arched doorway off to the side at one end of the church opposite the main entrance.

It became known for its function: "the Leper Door." Through it, those whose leprosy made them outcasts in the community were admitted to church services, but only in such a way that "the unclean" might not contaminate the upstanding churchgoers who entered through the main doorway.

After noticing the door on the run, I came back later to examine it and found that it had been bricked up. I was curious to know what had occasioned this change in construction: the understanding that leprosy was not all that contagious, in the era that ushered in multiple drug therapy for its control? Or perhaps a change of heart, the congregation rethinking its ostracism of the unfortunate sufferers of this Biblical disease?

When I first asked a church official about the door, I was told that the latter had occurred, that Christian mercy had overcome fear, and that repentant, large-minded parishioners had bricked up the door. But when I explored further, other facts emerged. In 1958, the leper colony that had formed near the station was moved to a "safer," more remote location. Thus the problem went away with the patients and the Leper Door could be bricked up, as it remains to this day.

As leprosy did a century ago, a new plague is ravaging Malawi and much of sub-Saharan Africa. The appalling effects of AIDS can best be summarized by this: In my first ten days operating in the Embangweni Hospital theater, I had not operated on anyone who was not HIV positive with the exception of two patients, and we were unsure of their status only because they had not been tested. Many of these people have stigmata of Kaposi's sarcoma lesions, every bit as much a mark of their condition as were the lost digits and facial features of the leprosy patients.

Leprosy patients had a disease that was chronic and morbid but at least not lethal in the majority of instances. Here, all patients with HIV and advanced stages of AIDS have a lethal condition. Perhaps the Leper Door might be reopened for the special admission of those with a far more serious plague than the one for which it originally was made?

With the AIDS epidemic sweeping Africa and the world, we might examine our own doors and who we admit through them. The Leper Door was bricked up because the people so stigmatized had been even further isolated. Perhaps the mortar should come out from the bricks if we are going to admit people living with AIDS fully into society for help and healing. Or perhaps we will continue to banish "the unclean," "the other," again and again.

Wherever I go, I am invited to view some group as "the other": lepers, Communists, women, Shiites, pagans, the bewitched, the HIV-positive. My response is always the same: "Ah yes, I see, these people are not at all like us. These people are us."

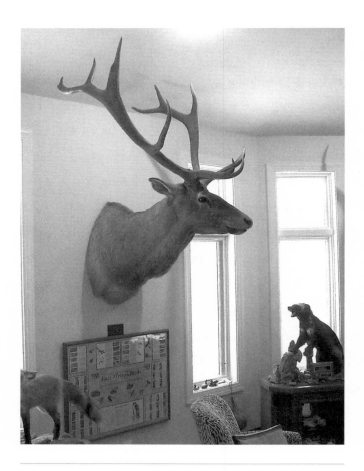

The game room of Glenn's Derwood, Maryland, home displays trophies and photos from his hunting expeditions and other adventures.

CHAPTER THIRTEEN

The Hunter-Gatherer and The Runner

AS A SURGEON, SAYS DR. CRAIG SCHAEFER, "YOU DON'T DO WHAT YOU do without having some confidence in yourself and some ego with regard to your abilities. Think of it as being an 'alpha male'"—leader of the pack, master of the situation.

The description fits Glenn, says his longtime friend Schaefer, not just in medicine but in two pastimes Glenn adores: hunting and running. An avid runner, Glenn has completed scores of long-distance races, including marathons on all seven continents and with each son. A self-described "hunter-gatherer" who savors hunting as a primal, natural pursuit, Glenn has stalked big game around the world and has dozens of taxidermic trophies (plus a freezer full of meat and fowl) to prove it.

Whether Glenn is practicing medicine in stripped-down settings, stalking an elusive beast or running an ultra-marathon, Schaefer says, the approach is the same. "Glenn chooses these fields that are not easy to be in," he says, "and drives himself to be the best he can be at them."

The lengthy accounts Glenn writes about hunting and running, like his accounts of medical exploits, are infinitely detailed and full of data. But there's something more in them as well. In the running diaries, he expresses a profound exhilaration from both the camaraderie with fellow runners and the individual triumph at the finish line. And in the hunting diaries, he conveys a peacefulness, almost a poetry; a reveling in the natural world as much as in the marksman's skills and kills.

The friendship began at GWU Medical Center. Craig Schaefer was a medical intern and resident, and Glenn was chief resident and an associate professor. Some thirty-five years later, veteran surgeon Schaefer says Glenn is "like family—akin to a brother to me and a close uncle to my children." Glenn places Schaefer in one of his most exalted categories of friendship: "not just a good buddy, but a hunting buddy."

Schaefer had gone hunting exactly once in his life when Glenn invited him out during Maryland duck season in 1982. From then on, the two have gone hunting regularly, all over the country for all sorts of game. Their hunts begat traditions: Virtually every Thanksgiving that he's in the country, Glenn joins the Schaefer family for dinner and the unpacking of Christmas decorations, followed by a weekend of duck and deer hunts.

Glenn's deep connection to hunting is fundamentally a connection to tradition, Schaefer believes. "Hunting is something he has done his entire life," he says, "more than medicine or travel or anything else." But Schaefer also sees Glenn's approach to hunting as all of a piece with the way Glenn navigates life:

Glenn views himself on a primitive level, as a hunter-gatherer, as he says. Hunting is a verification of his independence and his ability to handle problems, to think on your feet, come up with solutions and arrive at a positive outcome. With Glenn, that positive outcome can be anything from feeding and sheltering yourself on a hunt to fixing up your neighbor, literally. On a hunt, if you're tracking an animal and can't find your way back to camp, you have to find a way to survive. In the operating room, it's the same situation: You're trying to fix somebody's perforated ulcer, and the next thing you know, there's a hole in something that's not supposed to be there, and whatever the cause, you have to fix the problem.

The people you can go to when the chips are down have a proven record of thinking their way through those kinds of problems. They're the ones who are recognized as survivors. That's Glenn. He has the ability to take a lousy situation and make it good, not only in his professional life and his personal life but also in something like hunting. And in hunting, if he gets himself into a pickle, it becomes an adventure.

On a fall hunting trip with Schaefer and three others in the remote reaches of northern Quebec, Glenn brought down two big bull caribou, one with a rifle and one with an arrow from a high-powered bow. He spent hours in the tundra tracking caribou and doing what early American Indians called "counting coups"—showing stalking prowess by coming close enough upwind to the quarry to touch it with no intent to shoot. As the trip neared its end, he set out to track black bear with a fellow hunter named Harry, a journalist for an outdoor-sports television program.

After hours of hiking over tundra, looking for signs of bear and photographing scenery, "We realized our predicament," Glenn later wrote in his journal. "The sun was gone; we had circled swamps and featureless ridges; we were disoriented—we were lost." In the fading light, the two chose a lakeside spot where Glenn thought rescuers in a float plane might see them. Glenn took off his blaze-orange vest, pulled on a garbage bag in place of it, and hoisted the vest on a sapling as a signal flag. He and Harry tore off boughs to make a "spruce nest" that would raise them off the marshy ground. They tore off more boughs to fashion a roof and settled in for the night. "Even in these unplanned circumstances, the wonder of the wilderness is imposing," Glenn later wrote in his journal:

Shivering in the chill, and running through all the outdoor strategies for survival that we could think of did not preoccupy us so much that we did not marvel at the aurora borealis over our upturned faces or hear the warbling cry of the loon from the lake. It began to rain, and we could see steam rising from the spruce nest — leaking life energy into the barren ground.

Harry asked if I were a religious man . . . The spruce nest turned confessional, as he said he had never thought his life would end in hypothermia, but this was the penalty paid for a mistake in this unforgiving environment. He said goodbye to his wife and kids into my Dictaphone, then shivered violently as we piled more spruce boughs over the top of us curled up in some shelter from the wind but not the rain.

With dawn came heavy fog. We hunkered down to save energy until the fog began clearing at noon. Then I hiked to the top of one of the ridges to see if I could glimpse the lake our camp was on, and we began heading in the direction a float plane would take. After three hours, we heard it: a plane engine. The pilot Camil had spotted our blaze orange signal. Harry choked up at the arrival of this aluminum angel on floats, as it waggled its wings and landed into the nearby tundra lake. We walked back in silence to the lake where Camil told us, "We thought the bear got you."

Harry later wrote me an interesting letter about the value of this experience as a turning point in his life. On the outside of the envelope, his daughter Elizabeth had scrawled, "Thanks for saving my dad!"

After that outing, Glenn's Christmas present from Craig Schaefer's wife Carol was a battery-powered GPS unit (which he uses to this day). Thus began a new series of notations in Glenn's journals: the latitude and longitude coordinates of key stops on his travels.

"I think if Glenn could hunt 365 days a year, he would," Schaefer observes. "I've never seen him approach a hunt without the same enthusiasm, regardless of the difficulties—snowbound, mosquito-infested, whatever. Every time he goes out, it's like he's renewing himself."

Whenever possible, Glenn tacks a hunting adventure on to a mission, a conference or a lecture trip. Most autumns for the past dozen years, after the annual conference of the American College of Surgeons, Glenn and several surgeon friends have reconvened in Colorado for the opening of elk season. After a provisioning trip that Glenn has refined to an art—"without a list or helpers, total elapsed time of forty minutes, two giant overloaded grocery carts," he once crowed to his journal—the group takes horses and pack mules up snowy trails in the Rockies. At about twelve thousand feet, they make camp, living in a tent for five days of hunting.

Some years the hunters have shot several elk, then laboriously field-dressed and packed out the meat (consistent with Glenn's abject refusal to waste food). Other years no one even spots an elk. In either case, Glenn comes away with tales of adventure: about the time his shot knocked a bull elk off a cliff and he scrambled down a 1,700-foot vertical drop to retrieve the animal; or the time a packhorse reared and came down on Glenn's left leg, breaking it just weeks before he was to run two marathons (the Marine Corps Marathon in Washington, D.C., followed by the New York City Marathon).

Besides North America, Glenn has hunted on four other continents: in Venezuela for *pato real* (royal duck) and in Australia for buffalo; in Sweden for moose and in Micronesia for roe deer stag and feral hog. In the arctic mountains of Russia, he pursued bighorn snow sheep and giant brown bear; in Azerbaijan he was among the first Westerners admitted to hunt the Caucasus tur, an elusive goat-antelope prized for its scimitar-shaped horns. On international hunts where he cannot bring game home, he finds locals who can use it. From hunts closer to Derwood, he fills his basement freezer with meat and fowl that he loves to cook for friends. Taxidermic trophies from his hunts fill Derwood's "game room" and spill into the rest of the house.

Of all Glenn's hunts, the ones during medical missions in Africa come closest to satisfying him on every level, as hunter-gatherer and humanitarian, sportsman and anthropologist. Adding his sophisticated firepower to local villagers' spears, Glenn delights in bringing home nourishment for his

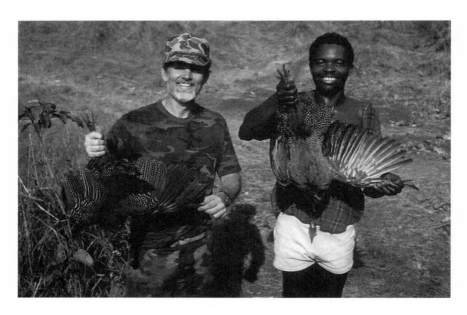

Glenn and Kongonyesi, a hunting companion from Assa, Congo, show off local kanga (guinea fowl) that they brought back for dinner.

patients, being provider as well as healer. And he loves how, in this activity, the tables are turned. In the operating room he is the expert and teacher, but in the bush he is the pupil, in awe of the tracking skills local hunters have honed over centuries as a matter of survival. "I am a highly skilled hunter by North American standards," Glenn once wrote, "and if I worked at it for years I might come up to one-tenth of the skill of my number-one hunting companion in Assa"—Jean Marco, son of the master "talking drum" carver Bule.

During one of Glenn's medical missions, Assa was preparing to host a large gathering of leaders from neighboring villages and, as host, was expected to feed those assembled. In an essay, Glenn described the hunting party he and Jean Marco led to provide meat for the feast "by subduing nearly one ton of humorless, vindictive, dangerous wild bovid—the Cape buffalo, known here as *nyati*."

The hunt began at 3:00 a.m. We had ten kilometers to cover to reach the Zara waterhole where nyati congregate in the dry season, and we needed to arrive fully a half hour before light in order to lay out strategy depending on what could be seen or scented. We stood in a circle in faint starlight, adjusting straps of knapsacks that held water flasks, snacks for a long day's excursion, skinning and dressing equipment in the event that we were successful, and a spare sleeve of heavy caliber bullets for my .375 Weatherby rifle.

Kongonyesi said the prayer for the hunt before we set out. It was simplicity itself, beginning with a hope for safety of all concerned, that we might see game, and that we might give a good account of ourselves in trying to secure food for those who will be needing it. Jean Marco set out in the lead with me immediately behind him, then the other hunters, the trackers and the bearers, about ten in all. Those at the rear carried the likonga, a venerable spear that had pierced many a buffalo when used in its best defensive position: its bronze head pointed at the charging buffalo, the end of its shaft planted under the heel of the spear-bearer who must make a desperate, last-minute scramble away as the buffalo impales itself on the strength of its own charge.

We cut through eleven-foot-tall elephant grass, then riverine jungle with thick, hanging liana vines; we waded streams up to our knees and sunk in mud crossing the marshland to the Zara waterhole. We covered the ten kilometers in just around an hour and waited for it to get just light enough to see without torches. Sitting in the dark, we could hear the screech of chimps in the tree cover and the heavy sloshing of large herbivores moving through the marsh. At one point we could hear the grunting, bawling and snort of Cape buffalo threats. Nyati was here. We were on time. I chambered a round.

At 5:30 a.m., the others remained seated as Jean Marco and I rose in the near-dark and walked to the slope leading down into the waterhole, screened by stands of grasses. Before we even got into the marsh, we heard sounds of running through the water course. Perhaps the herd had scented us. We came across a wide, trampled swath of a large group of hoof prints — evidently a very large herd. They may have moved out spontaneously or we had spooked them inadvertently, but they had given us the slip. For such a big and ugly animal, they can fade away as quickly and gracefully as a wraith.

The orange ball of the sun rose, sending dazzling streaks through the mist. As we advanced up out of the marshland, there was no trouble following the buffalo spoor. First we saw clods of mud, the buffalo shedding what they'd wallowed through in Zara. Later we could see rivulets of urine; a bearer who put a practiced toe in one of the rivulets reported the urine still was warm. The buffalo were easing away from us at about the same rate we were advancing — evidence that we had not spooked the herd, which is a good thing. Cape buffalo have a superb sense of smell, rather poor eyesight, and enough predatory cunning and stealth that they have been known to stalk the hunters who are stalking them. If this herd had moved off, having scented or sighted us, there might be a rear guard or a circling back of some of the beasts to have another look at us, to see what hunter was so audacious as to invade their turf.

A Cape buffalo tries to stay within a few kilometers of water, since he will have to visit it regularly to take in the thirty-five to forty liters of water that a big bull consumes in a day. It appeared that the buffalo were flanking a little hill and would probably arrive over the next ridge down into a river valley. A strategy was devised: Jean Marco and I would cut straight over the ridge, keeping watch of the wind direction, and try to go directly to the site where the buffalo most likely would be watering. The others in the group would continue to follow the buffalo tracks, in case they were taking a course other than the one we predicted.

When Jean Marco and I made it to the water, we heard grunting and splashing ahead on the other side of the screen of riverbank trees and underbrush. We slid into the forest cover and waited until the trackers and bearers joined us there. We waited for a second time as we heard the herd move off through the water and up the bank on the far side, then advanced upstream in order to cross higher than they had. When we crawled out from the riverbank margin, we could see a small funnel of dust almost a kilometer ahead of us marking the passage of the herd.

As the trackers and bearers continued to wait in the cover, Jean Marco and I went forward into the wind and at a perpendicular intercept to where we thought the herd might be in about half an hour, near a series of rocky ridges where we could look down from higher ground.

Jean Marco got to the ridge first and climbed up a small tree to look forward. He pointed in the distance to his left, and I eased forward nearly reaching the ridge. When Jean Marco came down from the tree, he advanced, but I didn't know where he was in front of me. I had crouched and was planning to sneak forward to the top of the ridge to look down into the next trough when I looked to the left and froze. A big bull buffalo was standing 125 meters to my left, with head back, nose up and both ears fanned in my direction. I was in the open and squatting with rifle across my left knee, but I did not move. The buffalo was clearly within range and standing in good position for a frontal shot at the neck and shoulder region. But I did not know where Jean Marco was, and I didn't know how many other buffalo might be around this one.

I soon learned. Moving from behind the buffalo were a series of perhaps six or eight buffalo ranging in size from calves up to large cows and one other bull. Single file, they came up behind the sentinel bull that appeared to be locked on me. Then the cows and calves gathered into a group and briskly trotted toward the ridge to my right where I presumed Jean Marco was.

The other bull came up behind the first one and stood in the same position and posture, both of them now polarized in my direction. For a moment I had an idea that I could take the first one and then quickly swing to the second and our hunt would be over and the larders would be filled. The buffalo looked frozen in position and time hung heavy. Then I realized there was a brisk breeze in my face which was coming directly from them. Their best sense was not helping them.

The second buffalo gave a snort and crossed behind the first and trotted off in the direction of the group that had moved on. The sentinel bull remained. I did my best to resemble a bush, crouched motionless without any cover anywhere around me, hoping the wind didn't change. I could not move to look at my watch, but we had been in this staring contest for some time when the horizon all around seemed to move. Heads down in a lumbering gait, buffalo appeared to my left, behind the sentinel bull, and to my right. They were all still upwind, but it suddenly occurred to me what had come of our strategy. Jean Marco had come up ahead of the herd and was probably on the ridge looking at the advancing beasts as they headed into the second trough. I, however, had come into the middle of the herd, and I would soon have buffalo on every side. And I was sitting, wide open, in their path.

I certainly could have zeroed in well on the big bull, but I had no way of knowing what would happen next, nor where any from our hunting party might be that could get swallowed up in the resulting melee. I stayed crouched, my toes tingling from lack of circulation. With occasional grunts and what sounded for all the world like burps, the buffalo herd moved toward the ridge. The big bull once again lined up on me with his nose held high and then ambled off following the herd. I waited for awhile before getting up. When I did so and scrambled up over the ridge, I saw Jean Marco coming toward me with a grin as if to say, "Seen any buffalo?"

For the third time during the hunt on this day, we allowed them to move off ahead of us. Then we resumed our tracking, and, staying close to Jean Marco this time, I resigned myself to another long hike. I had settled into a steady gait when I saw Jean Marco freeze in mid-stride. I stopped and saw, straight ahead, a big black body standing broadside with head raised and nostrils flared.

There was a low tree in front of me with a branch right across eye level. Slowly I raised the rifle to rest on the branch, and through the rifle scope, I recognized him: It was the big bull who had engaged me in the staring contest, now about 150 meters away. This time I knew where Jean Marco was, and I knew of no buffalo behind him. I flipped the rifle's safety catch, aimed just forward of the buffalo's shoulder and squeezed the trigger.

I didn't see what happened next as the heavy kick from the rifle lost the buffalo from the scope, but I heard what sounded like a solid hit. Then I heard the hammering of hooves but had no idea how many or in which direction, and could see nothing in clouds of dust in front of me. Jean Marco, frozen until the shot, ran to my left, and I followed. As he scrambled to the top of a big anthill to get a better view, I looked to my right and saw a large splotch of red but no buffalo. I ejected the spent shell casing and chambered a new round. Jean Marco silently pointed forward, jumped down from the anthill, and hit the ground on a run. I ran behind him until I saw what he had pointed at: on a grassy patch in the rocky ground, a large black body, motionless.

I ran to within ten meters of the front end of the buffalo, whose head was down. Coming up slowly, I did with my rifle barrel what Jean Marco's clan for centuries has done with a spear point to confirm a kill: I touched the animal's eye, and he did not blink. After the lethal shot, the buffalo had run perhaps five hundred meters. Circling around, I saw his legs drawn up beneath him, and the haunches and hams raked with claw marks that had healed in very prominent scars. I imagined the ferocity of that past encounter in which a lion had taken a ride on the backside of this bull. Nyati had gotten away from that far superior hunter to fall victim to this one.

We heard footfalls and saw the rest of our party running up. Kongonyesi came forward, touched the buffalo and spoke briefly. "What did he say?" I asked, and it was translated thus into my tape recorder: "We are very grateful that we were all spared. We are thankful that we have succeeded, and, once again, at least for now, we will not be going hungry." This was the benediction of a real hunter with respect for the hunted.

Within a few minutes the whole group had begun "breaking down" and loading up the beef. Suspended on poles carried on bearers' shoulders were highly prized parts: the stomach and other

During one of Glenn's medical missions, knowing Assa was preparing to host and feed a large gathering of neighboring village leaders, Glenn led a party to hunt nyati, the Cape buffalo. The bull Glenn shot—with hunting companions Neke, to Glenn's left, and Jean Marco to his right—yielded hundreds of pounds of meat.

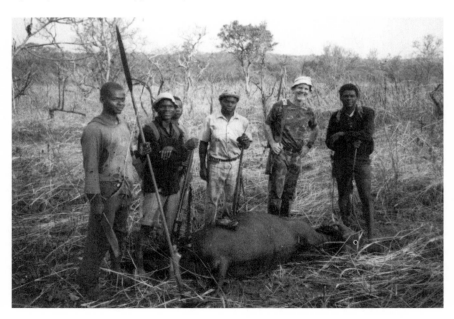

organs, and the head, which would feed a large family. Rib sections were threaded onto sharpened stick carriers, forequarters were balanced on heads, and large flank masses were lashed onto fresh-cut backpack frames. Each quarter had a hoof attached, which would be boiled to make a soup. The hide was used both as a wrapper to keep the meat until it could be further sectioned and also, with slits in it, as handholds for the shifting of the burden when the bearer was crossing streams. In contrast to wasteful tourist safaris where hunters may drop a ton of beef and saw off only the trophy horns to keep, every bit of this bull was loaded up for the long, rhythmic jog home.

Or almost every bit. I looked over the flattened grass and red-stained leaves where the buffalo had been so expertly disassembled and saw only one thing left behind. Catching up with Jean Marco, I attempted a passable French version of "Do we have everything?" and he nodded yes. I tried again: "But what about . . . " and I crooked my fingers at either side of my forehead. He got my meaning and this was his reply: "No one here eats the horns."

Glenn's friends in Assa do not understand it: Why does he run for miles through the bush when no animal is chasing him? They counsel him against this practice, and he notes their admonition in his journal: "*Dakta*, if you keep doing this, you never will have a fine, fat body."

While he has hunted for most of his life, Glenn took up running only in the late 1980s, inspired by his son Donald. Today, Donald Geelhoed, forty-four, is a shift sergeant with the Gainesville, Florida, police department, raising sons Andrew and Matthew and daughter Kacie with his wife, Kathy. Michael

Geelhoed, forty-one, is an assistant professor teaching physical therapy students at the University of Texas in San Antonio, raising twin sons Devin and Jordan with his wife, Judy. Neither Donald nor Michael shares Glenn's passion for hunting, but both are regular runners. So Glenn has fastened on running as one pursuit that he and his sons might all enjoy.

When he was a surgical resident at Harvard, Glenn took young Donald to the seventy-third running of the Boston Marathon. Glenn remembers the three-year-old, perched on his dad's shoulders, asking the obvious question as rain-soaked runners passed: "Why are these men doing this, Daddy?" As a teen growing up in Florida, Donald became a devoted runner, completing his first marathon at age seventeen.

During a Christmas 1988 visit with his father and Michael at Derwood, Donald was training for his next marathon with long laps around nearby Lake Needwood. On Christmas Eve, Glenn joined Donald for a mile. Within days, Glenn was adding miles and setting goals. On a summer 1989 stop in Greece, Glenn visited the stadium where the Olympics were born and ran its oval

In 2008, in San Antonio, Texas, Glenn and son Michael Geelhoed ran a marathon, then posed with Michael's wife Judy who ran a half marathon.

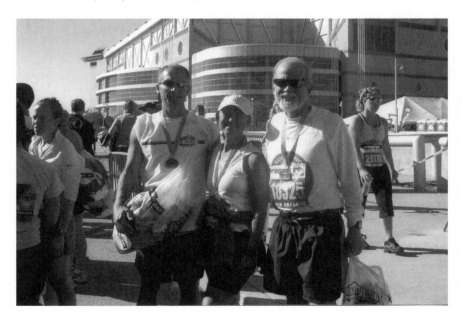

track. Crossing the finish line where the Athenian messenger Phidippides completed his run from Marathon to announce victory over the Spartans before falling over dead (thus giving the modern endurance race its name), Glenn resolved to attempt a marathon himself. The Marine Corps Marathon (MCM) he ran in Washington, D.C., that fall was the first race he'd ever entered, and he finished it in about 3:40—a qualifying pace, in his age range, for major races such as the Boston Marathon.

Glenn joined a Maryland runners club and became a regular entrant in the MCM, a tradition in the nation's capital. Over two decades he has run distance races in the shadows of Mount Everest and Mount Kilimanjaro, in Antarctica and Australia, Buenos Aires and Prague. He qualified years ago for membership in the Seven Continents Club, a society for runners who have completed marathons on every continent. He regularly runs what he considers short races, ten miles or ten kilometers, throughout the United States. And he has done eleven ultra-run events, multiples of a marathon, including races of roughly fifty-five miles in South Africa—from Durban to Pietermaritzburg—and in Wyoming and Montana, along the Bighorn River.

"My dad initially saw running as a way for us to connect, and then he took off with it, went full-fledged into it," Donald says. Donald's running career was interrupted dramatically in 2005 when, while training for a marathon to mark his fortieth birthday, he felt ill and was diagnosed with a heart-valve defect. Failure to correct it would lead rapidly to heart failure, Donald's cardiologist warned.

In fall 2005, Donald had a major operation to replace the congenitally defective aortic valve. And in 2007, running with police department colleagues as well as his father, Donald completed the Marine Corps Marathon. "I finished a respectable 4:11—nothing like my best marathon, but it was still better than I ever thought I would do," Donald says. "This was my exclamation point, my middle finger in the air to the disability of heart disease." He resolved to stick to half-marathons in the future but ran one last marathon with Glenn, in Florida in February 2008.

Several months later in Texas, Glenn and Michael ran the San Antonio Marathon, a race Glenn had run once before, in 1999. "The first

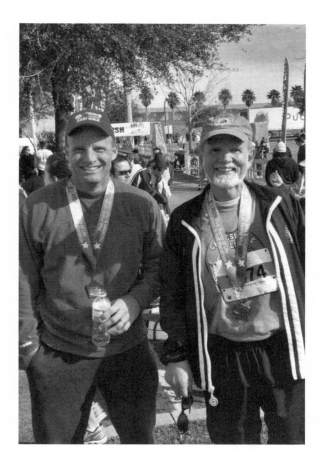

In Gainesville, Florida, in February 2008, Donald Geelhoed ran a marathon with his father.

time, my dad finished in about four hours; in 2008 he finished in about six hours, but he finished," Michael says. "It remains a way for him to stay in great physical shape. And it's like a lot of his pursuits: He doesn't go into any of them halfway. I think he just likes the experience of it all, swapping stories and being with other runners."

A runner Glenn met at the 1996 MCM has since become a friend and one of Glenn's personal heroes.

Joseph Patrick Aukward was born in November 1960, on the same day and in the same maternity ward as John Fitzgerald Kennedy Jr. He still jokes that mother Eileen, a first-generation Irish Catholic immigrant, was as excited to meet President Kennedy in the hospital as to welcome her new son, the sixth child of seven.

When Joe Aukward was six years old, his seventeen-year-old brother, Steve, a careful driver, had a couple of minor scrapes behind the wheel. Steve went in for a vision test, "and then the doctors wanted to test us all," Aukward recalls. "And I remember the doctor saying to my dad, 'Your little guy, he's the only other one of the children who has the condition.' "

The condition is retinitis pigmentosa, an uncommon, degenerative eye disease that generally runs in families and mostly affects males. As the disease progresses, gradual narrowing of peripheral vision causes partial vision loss in milder cases or, in more severe cases, complete blindness. Aukward matter-of-factly describes his retinitis pigmentosa as "advanced—I have only some light perception. I lost the balance of my usable vision between 1998 and 2000.

"But I was very lucky," Aukward insists. "I had a positive role model for dealing with this, my brother, and so I never had the sense that losing my eyesight was going to make my life less. And I lost my sight over more than thirty years, so I adapted in stages." At age six, with the onset of night blindness, he had to be more careful during evening hide-and-seek games in his New Carrollton, Maryland, neighborhood. Though he was a gifted football, baseball and basketball player through elementary school, by the time he was twelve his narrowing peripheral vision made it difficult to play ball sports, so he switched to running and clocked superb times in high school track events: the 440-yard dash in fifty-two seconds, the 880 in less than two minutes.

At seventeen, when Aukward moved to Baltimore to study accounting at a Catholic college, he could see well in only a twenty-degree range of central vision. He was so adept at operating with limited sight that "I could pass as being fully sighted very easily," he recalls. But as he met new people at college, he began revealing his condition and found friends who remained close as the disease progressed. And he kept up his athletic pursuits with the college's wrestling and cross-country track teams.

After graduating from college in 1982, Aukward took an accounting job with the U.S. Navy (where he has worked ever since, now in human-resource leadership). He bought a small house in New Carrollton near where he grew up. In a young-adult group at his church, he met Betty Volk. In early 1989, the two began dating; in late 1989, with his usable vision down to about three degrees, Aukward learned to use a cane. It has been in his hand for some of the happiest moments of his life: his 1991 wedding to Betty, who he calls "the love of my life," and the births of their children, Maria, Joseph and Michelle (who show no signs of retinitis pigmentosa).

But Aukward leaves the cane behind when he runs.

From youth, Aukward was what runners call "a natural," relaxed and fast. As he lost vision, what had been effortless became a struggle. Then in 1994 Aukward joined the U.S. Association for Blind Athletes and met a guide runner, Mark Lucas, whose advice made all the difference. "He said, 'I can tell you're fast and you have good endurance, but you're still trying to see. You have to stop that. You have to focus solely on running and leave the seeing to someone you totally trust to be your eyes and keep you safe.'" Aukward has done that ever since, with a committed cadre of guide runners that includes a journalist named Steve Nearman, a Marine named John Henry, an engineer named Daniel Will, and a physician named Glenn Geelhoed.

To run, Aukward holds in his right hand a tether, a shoestring-like cord about fifty centimeters long. The other end of the tether is held in the left hand of a guide runner, ideally, someone whose running skills match well with Aukward's. "When you're running well, you don't even feel the tether because it's slack," Aukward says. "If it gets taut, I know I'm going a little too far left." The guide runner's job is to match pace and stride with Aukward, give audible cues about the course and terrain, and generally free Aukward to focus on *how* he's running rather than where. "Not everybody embraces being a guide runner," says Aukward. "It's not about what the guide is feeling or wanting to do; it's about what the blind runner needs. They're truly selfless patriots."

With his guide runners, Aukward consistently runs a 5K race in about twenty minutes and a 10K race in about forty minutes. His personal best for a marathon is 3:36, run in 1997 in Chicago. Since 1998 he has competed

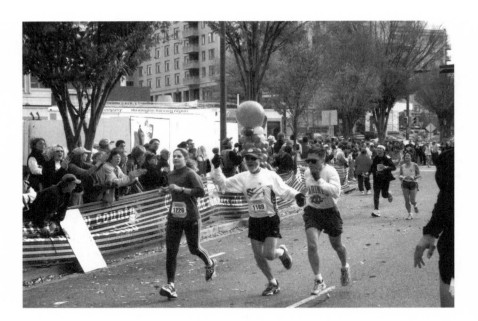

Glenn has completed numerous races, including marathons and half marathons, with his running buddy Joe Aukward. In 1995, the two crossed the finish line of the Marathon in the Parks in Montgomery County, Maryland.

internationally in Spain, Mexico, Canada and Greece. In 2000, ranked among the top dozen blind runners worldwide, he was training for the Paralympics, the premier event in the world for athletes with disabilities, to be held that year in Sydney, Australia. But in a 200-meter qualifying race, when guide runner Nearman ruptured his groin muscle coming around a tight curve and dropped the tether, Aukward came free and crashed into the track retaining wall. He suffered three broken ribs and disqualification from the Paralympics.

"It all worked out fine," Aukward says. During the time he was at home instead of in Sydney, daughter Michelle was conceived. And in 2004, Nearman again trained with Aukward to reach that ultimate goal: competing in the Paralympics, this time in Athens.

"My friend Joe is the single most positive person I have ever known," Glenn wrote in his journal. "I once ran a 5K race with him, a benefit for athletes with disabilities, and he was the first such runner to finish the race. And after he won, he went back to cheer on every further finisher he could hear coming into the home stretch. While others whine about what life has dealt them, Joe just keeps moving forward. He is a wonderful father and husband and a person of deep faith. And though Joe is blind, he sees people and situations more clearly than many sighted people I know."

From what Aukward could see before he went blind, he retains an image of Glenn: slender, bearded, smiling. Using software that reads written text aloud, Aukward follows Glenn's reports from medical missions and admires his friend's work among the world's poorest patients. But Aukward experiences Glenn chiefly as a running buddy who eagerly tests his own limits as an athlete and scrupulously describes everything along the course that he wishes Aukward could see.

Early in their friendship, Glenn and Aukward ran together in marathons in Boston, Baltimore and Washington, as well as numerous shorter races. But "since Joe is better than I am and twenty years younger, I might slow him down in races," Glenn told his journal. So lately they've met mostly for training runs. Even though the runs are fewer, "the friendship endures," Aukward says. When the American College of Surgeons gave Glenn a humanitarian award in fall 2009, Joe traveled to Chicago to join Glenn at the award dinner.

"Some people have a greater thirst for adventures and experiences in life," says Craig Schaefer. "Glenn is one of those. The twist of fate is, he has this degenerative process."

All his life, Glenn has had perfect eyesight, extraordinary visual acuity without any form of correction. That still is true in the left eye, so with both eyes open, as when driving or operating, there is no perceptible change. But in 2008, on a hunting trip, looking with his right eye through a rifle scope, Glenn experienced a blank spot just where the crosshairs met. A few weeks later, while he was at the motor vehicle bureau for a driver's license renewal, his right eye could not read the bottom line on the vision test.

Examinations at GWU and Baltimore's Johns Hopkins University found a microscopic lesion—seven microns across, about the size of a red blood cell—in the right eye's fovea, the dimple in the retina that is the center of the eye's sharpest, highest-resolution vision. Glenn noted the diagnosis in his journal: "chronic serous retinopathy, idiopathic." In lay terms, it's a condition whose cause is not known but that typically worsens over time.

Every three months since the initial diagnosis, Glenn wrote, "I have had both eyes examined in excruciating precision by retinal photography, then fluorescein angiography of a blinding light strobe. The chief of the retinal service declares it 'stable;' it has not resolved, but has shown no change in the repeated, big-ticket, all-day workups." The one compensation, Glenn wrote, is that the fluorescein retinal photography "makes for spectacular photos."

Hunting buddy Schaefer believes that "99 percent of hunters, faced with a disability like that, would say, 'That's it, I'm no longer hunting.' But Glenn likes it too much to quit. It's like his running: On the one hand he knows he's not a world-class athlete, but on the other hand, how many people his age run marathons? He relishes whatever accomplishments he's able to make."

In the end, the hunting and running and adventuring, along with the medicine, are Glenn's way of extracting maximum reward from every moment. He hopes good genes and habits might afford him a life as healthy and long as his father's. He has retrieved patients from the brink of death and has cheated it himself, but he knows that won't always be the case. He likes how that point is made in a painting he found in Malawi and described in an essay:

For the Malawian portrayed, everything seemed to have gone wrong on this day. He had gone out to get firewood and in the course of cutting the tree, he is charged by a lion. He takes refuge in the tree he has been chopping and crawls up out of the lion's reach successfully, only to encounter a green mamba, a deadly poisonous snake, sharing the tree's perch with him. If that isn't bad enough, the tree is beginning to sag under the earlier cuts he had made in the trunk, and it is his misfortune to be falling over a river. It is apparent that that river is also not unoccupied, and he will be landing as a near neighbor to a crocodile.

The painting's title, in the local Timbuku language, is IFA SITITHAWIKA, "Nobody Can Run Away From Death" or, more loosely translated, "Nobody Gets Out of This Alive."

It is perhaps good to be reminded that there is no difference between any of us and the fellow in the tree. Since we all share this common fate, our attention should be focused on the lives we lead and what we do to infuse them with meaning. What is important is not so much the end point of life as the content — what we do to lessen the burdens of others around us.

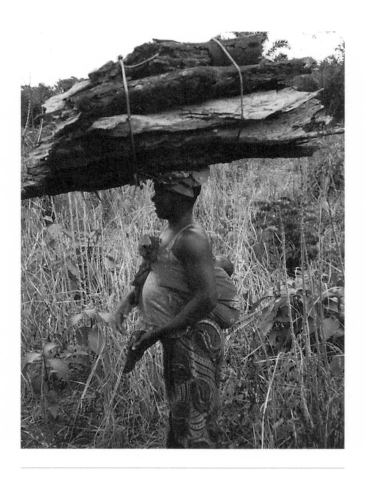

A woman in Assa, Congo, carries firewood on her head and a baby on her back.

CHAPTER FOURTEEN

Humility in Health Care

THE CASSAVA EATEN DAILY BY GLENN'S PATIENTS IN ASSA CONTAINED traces of cyanide, a chemical that encourages hypothyroidism. To make matters worse, the way Azande villagers prepared the cassava—soaking it in stagnant pools to soften the pulpy root—concentrated its cyanide content. Glenn suggested an alternative: Could the roots instead be soaked in the stream, where running water would wash the chemical away?

As much as villagers admired Glenn, they considered his suggestion witless: Who would put precious food in running water that might carry it away? *Zungu za wazungu*, they called his idea: "white man's madness."

The critiques were more sophisticated, but no less emphatic, when the scientific journal *Nutrition* published Glenn's findings from the Goiter Project. In a twenty-five-page paper in the journal's November/December 1999 issue, Glenn reached a provocative conclusion: that some effects of thyroid disorder actually helped the Congolese adapt to scarce resources, and treating the disorder removed that adaptive advantage. His paper sparked an unprecedented medical-ethics debate in the journal's pages.

Fifteen years after the iodine treatment program was launched, Glenn's paper described its results. Some four thousand Congolese were treated with long-lasting injections (in medical terms, "depot iodine"). After the injections, most patients' thyroid hormone levels returned to a normal range (the state called "euthyroid") and held at that level for several years. Many patients' goiters shrank dramatically or virtually disappeared after the injections (though for three dozen patients with particularly large goiters, Glenn operated to remove the growth, then gave iodine to inhibit re-growth). Women who had been treated with iodine bore children with no signs of cretinism. Three cretins who had been mute began talking; others began to draw or use tools for the first time. More babies were born, and fewer babies and mothers died during childbirth.

When forty village leaders were surveyed at the project's ten-year mark, they "unanimously reported remarkably positive changes in each of the individuals" who'd been treated, Glenn's paper noted. But controlling hypothyroidism also had upset a balance: The elimination of some problems had triggered others, the paper reported. The treatment program's intended, positive outcomes—increased health and fertility—had had unintended, negative consequences:

- As villagers in Assa regained energy, Glenn reported, they became more active, hungrier, and unable to get by on the cassava-based diet as before. "More of the forest surrounding the small village was slashed and burned for increased garden plots, and people walked farther for food, firewood and water," he wrote in the paper.

- "Not only has fertility increased dramatically, but elimination of neonatal cretinism has caused the stillbirth rate to plummet," Glenn wrote in the paper. As a result, he reported, just eight years after the start of the treatment program, the population of the area had doubled. "Compounds have become villages and villages have become crowded."

- The rapid population growth caused "considerable degradation of what had been a typically luxuriant tropical forest ecology," Glenn wrote in the paper. "Four streams, no longer adequate, are now also polluted. Latrines had been built, but are now crowded past capacity."

♦ As growth further strained the area's meager resources, "some families are sending forth migrants" to try to find work, Glenn wrote. The nearest city, and even the nearest transportation to reach a city, was far away, he noted. And if those who ventured forth did return, he wrote, "they may bring back deadly social diseases, as one has already."

Glenn's paper concluded with two verdicts on the project: a simple one from Zandeland's leaders and a more penetrating one of his own.

In Assa and neighboring villages, Glenn wrote, the people "are uniformly appreciative of the medical-intervention program" in terms of its effects on individuals' wellbeing. At the same time, he wrote, villagers complained about changes in their community—pollution, crowding, hunger—without perceiving them as related to the changes in their health.

To Glenn, the relationship was clear, and reason to reflect more broadly on the role of medical intervention. For the villagers whose hypothyroidism was controlled, the Goiter Project had "a very obvious and overwhelmingly positive beneficial consequence," he wrote. However, "when viewed from the perspective of the society of which these individuals are a part, the negative consequences of medical intervention . . . become more prominent." For centuries, he reasoned, hypothyroidism might have been nature's way of helping people survive in marginal habitats by living low-energy, low-consumption lives. When iodine injections changed that balance, the healthier inhabitants of Zandeland outstripped its capacity to support them.

Glenn's paper offered the Goiter Project as "an instructive lesson in both the potential and limitations of medical intervention in a complex human social problem."

Dr. Michael Meguid, like Glenn, had done his surgical residency at the Brigham and worked with Dr. Francis D. Moore. Meguid went on to pursue research and surgical specialties relating to cancer, metabolism and nutrition. And in 1985 he founded the journal of which he remains editor-in-chief, *Nutrition: The International Journal of Applied and Basic Nutritional Sciences.*

When Meguid received Glenn's paper, he initiated the journal's customary peer-review process. He sent the manuscript to three reviewers with relevant expertise, including one in Africa. He asked for the reviewers' appraisals of the paper's content and their opinion on whether it should be published. When the reviews came back, they reflected such dissenting opinions, so passionately expressed, that Meguid saw no "consensus opinion concerning the scientific and overall merit of the work." And so began an expanded process of review, commentary and response that, when published, consumed nearly a fifth of the 188-page journal.

As Meguid described the process in an editorial, he next sent the manuscript "to three additional reviewers carefully selected to cover the topics of endocrinology, African affairs and medical ethics, because it is in these three areas that the differences of opinion emerged. The views of the three subsequent referees, alas, did not resolve the controversy. Instead they reflected the same spectrum of diverse opinions as did the first three reviewers. The basic issue of those in opposition is that this study was 'unethical, should never have been performed and, furthermore, despite being performed, should not be published,' but these were minority opinions.

"After I had initially reread the lengthy manuscript, my thoughts reflected in part the spectrum of thoughts expressed by all six reviewers," Meguid wrote. "All had expressed legitimate viewpoints. However, in the end I feel that is it not an editor's job to practice censorship." So Meguid recruited more reviewers, physicians and scientists whose expertise ranged from medical ethics and surgery to the history of iodine-deficiency disease. He then published a journal special report that included Glenn's original paper, reviewers' commentaries on it and, in what he called "an unprecedented step, the final word in the form of reflections and analysis by Geelhoed."

Reviewer Dr. Jeremy Sugarman, a Duke University MD and medical ethicist, questioned whether participants in the Goiter Project had enough information about its possible risks and benefits to give truly informed consent. He questioned whether the project met a medical-research standard called the principle of beneficence, which "requires that benefits to subjects are maximized and potential harms minimized . . . In this case, it seems that several of the harms experienced by the subjects were predictable," Sugarman wrote, referring to the increased fertility that led to village crowding and the villagers' increased appetites, which led to hunger.

At the least, Sugarman wrote, "The harms described by Geelhoed should have been anticipated and an appropriate infrastructure developed to deal with them." But given the potential for these outcomes, he asked, "should this experiment have been done in the first place? . . . What has happened to this unfortunate group of persons that briefly 'tasted' a euthyroid life? How can they make sense of a short-term intervention that caused societal devastation? Who has apologized? And how can we ensure that this sort of thing does not happen again?"

A second reviewer was medical ethicist Dr. Robert W. Daly, MD, of the State University of New York at Syracuse. Daly wrote that he appreciated Glenn's interest in studying and treating hypothyroidism in Zandeland: "To acquire knowledge that provides the basis for healing and to improve the health of persons, both individually and collectively, are goals worth pursuing," he wrote. But despite some benefits from the work of Glenn and the Goiter Project, Daly said he had "serious concerns about the ethical propriety of the author's activities."

Daly questioned whether the project met international ethical standards for medical research involving human subjects, especially mentally impaired ones like the cretins. And he suggested those who ran the Goiter Project should have anticipated "the untoward biological and social consequences of providing depot iodine to four thousand Azande. The benefits and risks, individual and collective, of successfully treating hypothyroid persons with depot iodine were well known fifteen years ago. It should not have taken a great leap of scientific imagination in the 1980s to realize what would happen to the Azande and their habitat when they became euthyroid."

Daly was particularly critical of Glenn's statement that Goiter Project participants didn't make a connection between improvements in their health and problems in their environment. He characterized Glenn as "withholding" information about that connection, and he called that "simply wrong, morally blameworthy, a clear example of bad faith, a violation of human trust."

Editor Meguid assigned a third reviewer, British surgeon and ethicist Dr. John MacFie, MD, to "attempt to find common ground" between Sugarman's and Daly's views and Glenn's. The best MacFie could do was a few even-handed generalizations: If the villagers were "voluntary participants in (Glenn's) study, then arguably the study was ethical because there was no exploitation," he wrote. And the fact that medical interventions "have profound social consequences . . . does not render them unethical. It simply emphasizes our responsibility to consider long-term effects on populations."

In the closing editorial commentary where Meguid gave Glenn "the final word," Glenn's remarks were by turns dryly critical, painstakingly detailed and frankly philosophical.

Glenn faulted the *Nutrition* special report for including too many "minority dissenting views . . . Whereas alternative views complimenting the study are not represented." He contended that the reviewers lacked sufficient understanding of his work in particular and the developing world in general. And he suggested that critics' real problem with his study was the uncomfortable truth it revealed: that health-care interventions in poor countries "may have caused as much trouble as we have allegedly cured, but we have turned our backs when the later data came in because those unwanted consequences are either 'not my job' or 'outside our expertise.'"

Neither he nor anyone else in the Goiter Project had set out to "study experimental subjects" as reviewers claimed, Glenn wrote. "This was a treatment program, begun cautiously in a remote setting. The population itself had made repeated and insistent requests [for treatment], worked out with all the implications that could be foreseen in long sessions of the council of village elders." When the elders were warned that less-lethargic people would need more to eat, they replied that those people also would be able to grow and gather more food. When villagers were told that iodine treatments would increase fertility but that family-planning assistance could control it, "there was a clamor for the former and few takers for the latter," Glenn wrote.

When planning the treatment program, "the putative 'downside' may have

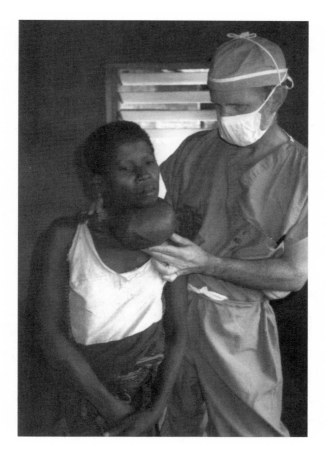

Glenn examines a Goiter Project patient in Assa. In late 1999, the scientific journal Nutrition *published Glenn's findings from the Project and his provocative conclusion: that some effects of thyroid disorder actually helped the Congolese adapt to scarce resources, and treating the disorder removed that adaptive advantage. His paper sparked an unprecedented medical-ethics debate in the journal's pages.*

---

lurked as a concern in the opinion of First-World observers," Glenn wrote. "But the population at Assa continues to think of the program as one of the most beneficial interactions they have ever had with any outside source of aid."

Glenn suggested it was not reviewers' place to second-guess the village elders who "considered, discussed and repeatedly pleaded for the institution of a health-care program to address especially the issue of what they saw as a social tragedy—the birth of insufficient numbers of children, and quite a number of them blighted by cretinism." He was particularly eager to answer the reviewer claim he found most distressing: that he had treated these patients without explaining to them how the healthier, bigger population could strain village resources.

"The claim," he wrote, "is that this group was studied, we found interesting consequences, and then abandoned them to their fate, possibly worse off than they might have been had they been not treated." Not true, Glenn insisted. Goiter Project administrators made "as full a disclosure, in Assa and elsewhere, of the secondary social consequences" of treatment as of its individual health benefits, he said. Nonetheless, villagers begged for the treatment. It was clear, Glenn wrote, that "they would rather discount almost any long-term ill in a setting in which they find immediate reward"—relief from strangling goiters, and babies born free of cretinism.

Goiter Project personnel tracked every patient in treatment and continued the follow-up study for years after, specifically "to determine the late consequences" both to individuals' health and to village life, Glenn wrote. After he and other Westerners left the area, the iodine injection and monitoring program was continued by the local health aides they had trained.

Glenn repeated a reviewer's question about whether his study should have been done at all, and then rephrased it: "Do we not know enough to act on that knowledge and predict the results, good and bad, of medical intervention? In my opinion, clearly not . . . A simplistic approach always arises from the impulse 'This much we know for sure, and this, at least, is one thing we can do!' A conclusion I draw from the data . . . is that life is never quite so simple and that we should not proceed on the basis of what we hold to be clearly self-evident, without a culturally sensitive perspective of consequences both seen and unforeseen."

With wording as genteel as he could muster, Glenn rejected the reviewers' perspectives as coming from "a First-World setting, once removed from both the report and the reality of those with much more urgent dilemmas and who seek help of a real and sustainable type." Such misperceptions, he suggested, were what caused culturally insensitive, narrowly focused, "vertical" health-care programs to be imposed, and to fail, in the developing world. And it would be those "silo" programs, he wrote, to which the reviewer's question might properly be directed: "How can we ensure that this sort of thing does not happen again?"

Like the Goiter Project itself, Glenn's study of the project was "undertaken with good intentions," Glenn wrote. When initial study data showed remarkable treatment successes, he was gratified. But when later data revealed more complex and even negative outcomes, he valued that knowledge as well. His study and the *Nutrition* exchange about it were a part of what he deemed a lesson well learned: that "humility in health care compels us to loiter long enough past our triumphs to be observant and honest . . . and to publish the downside along with the early victory statements."

Glenn's journal entry for July 22, 1998—the final day of his final trip to Assa—recorded some of what was accomplished during the visit: "Twenty-one major surgical operations under general anesthesia . . . Forty-seven dental extractions under local anesthesia . . . Eighty kilograms of pharmaceuticals and surgical instruments delivered . . . Eleven medical personnel trained or encouraged . . . " There was little left to do beyond one traditional, parting ritual: Just before he flew back to civilization, Glenn always removed the battered running shoes he had worn on the trip and bequeathed them to some unshod citizen.

A parade of capering children and tearful adults escorted him to the airstrip. When the Cessna had landed and the propeller-driven dust had settled, Glenn climbed into the copilot's seat.

"I fastened my seatbelt and opened the side window to shake more hands and to wave," he wrote in his journal. "When I looked up at the end of the turnaround part of the airstrip, there stood the old leper, with his unblinking face staring over at the plane, leaning on his stick, barefoot with only a few stubs of toes. It had taken a lot of time and effort for him to hobble down this far. As pilot Brad was about to shout 'Attention! Clear prop!' Jean Marco

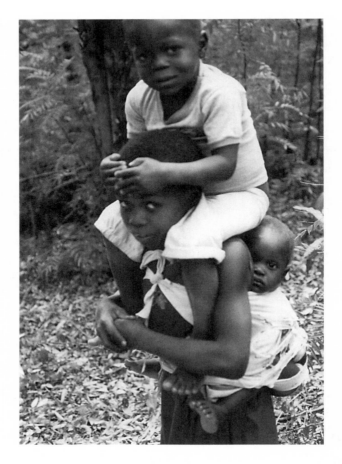

In Assa as in neighboring Congolese villages, older children care for younger ones while their parents are busy farming, hunting, gathering and cooking.

came around to the window to be the last to shake my hand.

"I looked away from the window and down at my feet. I loosened my seatbelt and darted down to the floor as Jean Marco waited with his hand outstretched. When I popped back up to retighten my belt, I reached out to Jean Marco and said, 'Today I do not walk; I will no longer need these.' And pointing to the old man, I dropped my shoes in Jean Marco's hands. Except for the old man, whose facial expression never changes, they were all crying. They were not alone."

Within weeks after Glenn's departure, expatriates were evacuated after rebels marched on the capital Kinshasa and overran Assa and its neighbors. The ensuing civil war would last more than five years and claim some three million lives.

A year after the *Nutrition* special issue, Glenn was featured in a publication of a very different sort: *George*, the magazine John F. Kennedy Jr. launched as a splashy mix of politics, celebrities and social issues. The October 2000 edition announced Glenn as one of *George's* "Citizens of the Year," people chosen for outstanding contributions in various fields of endeavor. The photo in *George*, shot during Glenn's mission to Ladahk, showed him against a dramatic backdrop: storm-darkened skies above hillsides lit by the sunset and rows of whitewashed *stupas*, mound-like shrines bearing the remains of Buddhist monks.

"Starting in medical school, Glenn W. Geelhoed's passion has been to provide help wherever there are too few doctors and there is too much illness," the accompanying article said. "So, though he has a day job—as a professor of surgery and of international medical education at George Washington University Medical Center —Geelhoed finds more fulfillment moonlighting as a medical missionary . . . Often operating solo, without organizational support, Geelhoed recruits students and other doctors to join him; most return again and again."

As for what drove his work, the article quoted Glenn's simple explanation: "I'm an American; I've been on the receiving end of a whole lot of advantages and have not even paid back the interest."

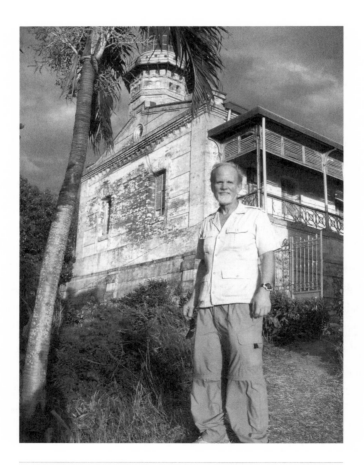

*On repeat medical missions to the island of Luzon, the Phillipines,
Glenn likes to show mission team members around his favorite local
sights including the Cape Bojeador Lighthouse.*

CHAPTER FIFTEEN

Hither by Thy Help

"COME, THOU FOUNT OF EVERY BLESSING." THE HYMN, WRITTEN BY AN eighteenth-century British preacher, had been one of Glenn's favorites since childhood. Its second stanza begins with a line that the world traveler has made his own: "Here I raise mine Ebenezer, 'Hither by thy help I'm come.'"

The lyric refers to an Old Testament story in the first book of Samuel. The Israelites had suffered a crushing defeat by the Philistines, with many lives lost. Then later—only after they sought God's help—the Israelites vanquished the same foe at the very same location. To mark that battle site, the prophet Samuel placed a large memorial stone, which he named Ebenezer, Hebrew for "stone of help." Through Christian history, any talisman reminding believers that they live only "by God's help" has come to be called an Ebenezer.

Virtually everywhere he has traveled since the 1968 mission to Nigeria, Glenn has carried some bit of paper bearing the single word Ebenezer. First it was a 3-by-5 card with Old English lettering cut out and pasted on, laminated to make it sturdier. When that card began to disintegrate after years of travels, Glenn retired it and made replacements with whatever was handy: the stub of a museum entry ticket, the back of an airline boarding pass.

It has become Glenn's quiet ritual, in thanks for God's protection, to unpack the Ebenezer first when he reaches a destination. He places it on a desk or nightstand when there is one. But just as often, he places it in the fold of a mosquito net, or on the floor by a sleeping mat. Sometimes he packs it for departure to go forward to the next stop; sometimes he leaves it behind as a sort of "Geelhoed Slept Here" marker.

Since college, Glenn has carried the same style of thin, fifty-two-week date-book from the London stationer Smythson of Bond Street, with perforated, tear-off corners so the book opens easily to the current week's page. When Glenn begins a new week on the road, he places the torn-off page corner next to the Ebenezer. He chuckles to imagine what meanings have been ascribed to those little paper shrines in the places he has left them: in a hotel suite in Mumbai and a yurt in Kazakhstan, at Uhuru Point on Mount Kilimanjaro, in an ice cairn in the Antarctic, on a giant lily pad in the Amazon River.

Glenn's religious philosophy is rooted in Bible basics: *Love your neighbor as yourself*; treat others as you would be treated. He does not broadcast publicly what he is happy to explain quietly, that medical missions are his way of living out his faith. But he begins to lose patience if pressed for sectarian specifics: Does his commitment and skill as a physician come from a particular god, a particular faith? If he heals in the name of his beliefs, shouldn't he share those beliefs with patients?

"My religious motivation is Christian because that's where I've come from," Glenn once wrote. "I had the upbringing I had, and I couch my beliefs in terms of it. But my religious motivation is no more or less valid than that of the great majority of my friends—people I admire greatly for their humanity and their spirituality—who are Shi'a or Hindu or Buddhist. My faith is not about going to bring someone out of darkness into the light. Rather, I go to find out what light others might shed on my own darkness."

The doctor of philosophy degree that Glenn completed in 2004 was rather beside the point. Over decades, he had studied the world's great thinkers, mined doctrines and philosophies, to develop his own worldview. He constructed it between what always had been the two poles of his existence, the sciences and the humanities. He tempered it with everything he had gleaned from a wide world of experiences. And he centered it on a conviction about what the rich, developed world owed to the poor, developing world.

"People like me just happen to be beneficiaries of a society that we had little part in making," he once wrote. "People in the developing world are on the front side of something that's only beginning. So what are we going to do about that? Isn't there an obligation? I believe in the 1980s the prevailing notion was, 'I don't have any real obligation to fix somebody in another part of the world unless it's going to come back to bite me.' But the 1990s saw us begin to reconsider that. And in the new millennium, I believe it really is changing."

⸙

The late Dr. Tim Harrison, the colleague who first brought Glenn to Assa, was himself the son of a medical missionary. Starting in 1909, Tim's father, Dr. Paul Harrison, spent most of a half-century working throughout the Arabian Peninsula for the Presbyterian Church of America (PCA).

The PCA's Arabian mission efforts included evangelism, education and medical outreach. Paul Harrison devoted his talents to the latter two, founding hospitals, providing care and establishing one of the first medical schools in the region. In overwhelmingly Moslem cultures where Christians faced rejection and even persecution, Dr. Paul was respected and admired.

As Glenn tells the story that Tim shared with him, Paul Harrison once came before PCA officials to report on his work. He listed all that had been achieved in medical treatment, training and education. But church officials were looking for other information. *How many souls have you saved?* they asked. *How many decisions for Christ have come from your ministrations?* Dr. Paul's answer was as intentional as it was brief: "Only Allah knows."

Glenn's philosophy is much the same. A tireless recorder of data, he can reel off statistics about the bodies he has treated: eighteen hernia repairs during one South Sudan mission, fifty-seven thyroidectomies during one week in the Philippines. He knows that when he cures patients, their hearts are touched as well. But their souls he considers their inviolable personal property, subject to their own choices and not for him to claim or judge. He will pray with and for anyone who requests it. He will not take sides in denominational tussles. He will not proselytize—and his agreement not to

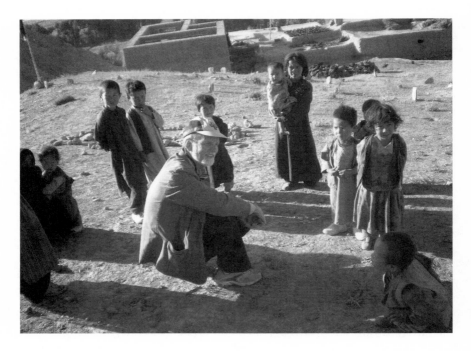

Glenn visits with local children during a mission to Afghanistan. He is allowed to work there, and in China, Chad and most of the Middle East, on condition that he not proselytize. Twice in recent years, volunteers Glenn has worked with in Afghanistan have been killed by militants who accused them of trying to spread Christianity.

is a precondition of being welcomed in such nations as Afghanistan, Nepal, Chad, Somaliland and China as well as most of the Middle East.

Glenn knows that breaking that agreement would risk expulsion, or worse. Days after he finished a 2008 mission in Kabul, Afghanistan, drive-by shooters killed Gayle Williams, a volunteer Glenn had worked with in Kabul, because they believed (mistakenly, Glenn says) that she had given Christian literature to Muslims. In August 2010, when ten medical aid workers in northern Afghanistan were gunned down by Taliban insurgents who accused the workers of spying and trying to spread Christianity, the news brought Glenn to tears. Among the dead was Cheryl Beckett, with whom he and Gayle had shared both medical and training projects and scenic hikes in the hills around Kabul.

Glenn's nonsectarian approach puts him at odds with organizations whose mission includes both evangelism and medical service. That has cost him some alliances, access to some grants and donations, but Glenn doesn't lose sleep over it. When he's tending a gravely ill patient, he is confident that all the prayers ascending—his own and others from any tongue or creed—are equally assured of a hearing.

_____

While Glenn personally bankrolls a healthy share of mission costs, his teams also draw important support from religious groups and individuals. For flights into remote locations, Glenn charters planes from Mission Aviation Fellowship and Africa Inland Mission Air, Christian-backed flight operations that transport medical, relief and missionary personnel. Mission team members find lodging in church-affiliated guest houses. Medicines and supplies come from organizations such as Medical Assistance Programs International, a Georgia-based Christian charity that has sent more than $1.75 billion worth of goods to medical missions since 1954. Faith-driven groups and individuals take it upon themselves to become what Glenn fondly calls "scroungers," collecting and donating much-needed supplies.

From his experiences throughout the developing world, Glenn feels confident making certain generalizations: that governments tend to be self-serving, short-sighted and corruptible; that militaries are fickle, customs officials are grasping and bureaucracies are unresponsive; that NGOs are often well-meaning but self-satisfied and paternalistic. When it comes to religious entities, though, Glenn's judgments are mixed. There are many faith-driven people and projects that he admires but also some he considers misguided, unworthy, even ridiculous.

He met an example of the former in Chico, California: "scrounger" Janice Walker and her surgeon-husband, David. And he wrote about the latter from Malawi, in an archly worded essay on "the phenomenon known as JJ—Junk for Jesus."

Somewhere in the world right now, there are teams of people scavenging everything that has outlived its usefulness in the developed world. After it has been rendered useless by a critical missing part, it is trundled into a big box and shipped to a center where it can bless the developing world—with no hope of ever functioning or ever encountering anyone who can repair it with the missing part that has doomed it to trash in the first place.

With noble but naïve intentions, some devout citizens in the First World have insisted that people here in Malawi should get everything that we have—if only a generation later, and after it has broken. The small, nettlesome fact about these donations is that shipping junk to the far side of the world in fact ends up benefiting only the First-World donors and burdening the "ungrateful" beneficiaries.

Hanging on a supply-room wall in the hospital here, there are four good-looking endoscopes. Nary a one of them works since they are fiber-optic and chip-containing, and the reason they were discarded in the first place is that they were broken. They could not be repaired in a First-World setting just crawling with equipment company reps and repairmen and parts stocks on the Internet. Out here, they are quite expensive decorative wall hangings.

A United States-based religious aid group sent the endoscopes. They were shipped in a cargo container (at considerable cost) along with other irreparably broken equipment, as well as medications that the Malawian health ministry will not allow to be used because they are past expiration date. It fell to local hospital officials to deal with all this very expensively transported medical waste. They threw the drugs into the river (with whatever environmental consequences that had on the precious Lake Malawi). The broken instruments went on display or gathered dust. The container went to a landfill. So much for the "generous donation" foisted upon these needy people.

On hospital rounds this morning, I looked around at the pastiche of brightly colored, crocheted woolen bed covers. I thought of the hundreds and thousands of church women across the American Midwest and South who have spent endless hours of ladies' circles crocheting these rather attractive and useful items. They might never even remotely imagine the settings in which their homemade contributions are being used—but they do get used, as items like these are hard to go wrong. However, make me a donation of a computerized, tomographic, laser-guided imaging unit, and I can assure you without looking that it is not working, will not be made to work, and never will work in the developing world. It will constitute a storage problem, even if it makes for an imposing backdrop for the donor photograph that will be sent back home.

At a hospital where I've worked in South Sudan, the hugely impressive anesthesia machine has more bells and whistles than any I have seen in the United States from which it came. Three consecutive teams have been sent out to try to get it to work but have been unable to resurrect it from the reason it was sent out to begin with: as a relatively new, very modern "lemon." The last I knew, the anesthesia machine, covered with a plastic tarp, was being used as *a side table. Beyond that, its benefits were just two: the hundred-thousand-dollar charitable write-off it allowed its First-World donors, and the payment collected by the shipper who jettisoned this shiny load of JJ on the far side of the world.*

Janice Walker organizes aid shipments that are manifestly not JJ. In 2004, with her children grown and her ear-nose-and-throat-surgeon husband, David, busy with patients, Janice was looking for "something to do that could make a difference in the lives of others." She inquired about volunteering with a local non-profit, Project S.A.V.E. (Salvage All Valuable Equipment). When she learned the project was near collapse, instead of becoming a volunteer, she took over as director.

Project S.A.V.E. collects medical and dental supplies and equipment from hospitals, clinics, professional organizations and individuals. Then its all-volunteer staff sorts, packs and ships the medical supplies, along with other necessities, to needy communities around the world. In the past six years, the project has expanded its shipments to thirty-five countries and has sent enough goods to fill sixty twenty-foot containers.

One of the first shipments Janice oversaw was to the Philippines island of Mindanao, to support the work of medical missionary Dr. Allan Melicor. In gratitude, Melicor invited Janice and David to visit. When they did, Janice recalls, "I spent much of the week weeping for joy to see the difference our goods made in this little hospital." David pitched in on patient care with other visiting doctors, Glenn among them. Once Janice heard Glenn's "bigger than life" stories of the missions he led, the two agreed to stay in touch and see how each could support the other's work.

One particular e-mail exchange with Janice convinced Glenn she was a kindred spirit.

On several medical missions, Glenn had worked with Stephne and Harry Bowers, a Christian missionary couple ministering to widows and orphans in Soddo, Ethiopia. So Glenn was pleased to see Janice's e-mail describing what Project S.A.V.E. had rounded up to send to the couple: "literally

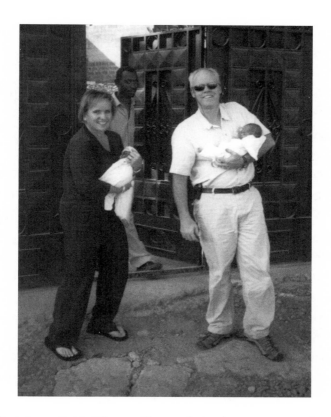

On medical missions to Soddo, Ethiopia, Glenn worked with missionaries Stephne and Harry Bowers, whose projects include ministering to widows and orphans. In 2008 when a mother died after bearing twins, Glenn accompanied the Bowerses to an agency that would place the babies with adoptive parents.

hundreds of dollars of new and used clothes for the orphanage . . . probably 100+ pairs of new shoes . . . lots of brand new baby clothes," plus diapers, food and clinic equipment.

Then came the bad news, in a message Stephne Bowers sent from Addis Ababa: "We are struggling to get the long-awaited container through customs. Since [the date when] precious friends gathered and filled the container . . . the government made changes regarding import laws and our duty-free status was adjusted before our helpless eyes! In order for us to get the container's content (which would feed and clothe so many of the poor in the south), customs is expecting us to pay US$7,000 in penalties for second-hand clothing, which is against the law to import. We watched 350 kilograms of clothing and shoes being burnt, while naked children watched from the other side of the fence! There is not much to be done in the flesh, so we are trusting the Father for His divine intervention . . . "

Angry and incredulous, Janice e-mailed the news to her volunteers and friends. "I cannot believe they burned the clothing and shoes," she wrote. "How can any government be so callous? It just sickened me."

"Some lessons we learn while doing this project are hard to take," Janice admitted. But this one did not shake her faith and only hardened her resolve. Immediately she went to work, rounding up donations to help cover the customs fees, figuring out how to head off problems with future shipments. Stephne and Harry Bowers asked Ethiopian government officials for one more meeting, to plead for the container's release.

Some ten days later, Stephne's e-mail to Janice was exultant: "IT IS HERE!!! The container's content arrived yesterday morning early from Addis and all the items were stacked high on [a truck]. It took me and ten guys all morning to unload. Then I sorted and organized the rest of the afternoon . . . I stand amazed at the hearts and hands of so many who donated and gave so very generously!" Though a quarter of the donations had been destroyed or diverted, the rest made it through.

Glenn congratulated Janice on the success. He told her his mission teams had many similar encounters with bureaucracy, some ending well but others in frustration. He spoke ruefully of how his mission personnel were treated in some countries: not as collaborators to be appreciated and thanked, but as rich targets to be manipulated and milked.

After enough encounters like that, a few team members inevitably come to Glenn downcast and ready to quit. The needs are too great and the systems too broken, they tell Glenn, *This is hopeless. There is nothing we can do for these people.*

Glenn's refusal to believe that is the sum and substance of his faith.

He rejects such lost-cause thinking as "the ultimate self-fulfilling prophecy." He insists that some good comes from even the smallest act of giving.

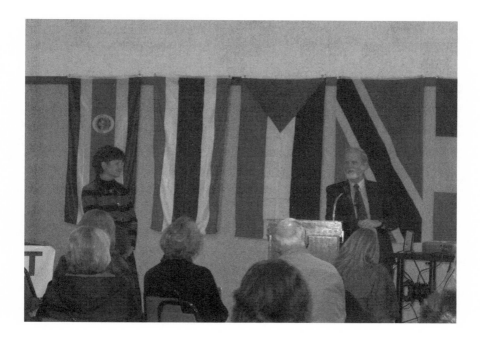

At a Chico, California, presentation organized by Project S.A.V.E. director Janice Walker (left), Glenn showed photos from the many medical missions where patients benefited from the supplies provided by groups like Project S.A.V.E.

He clings to the childhood catechism that declared him "saved to serve." And he feels morally obliged to help even when helping seems fruitless, thankless. It is this spirit in particular—loving a cause that others deem lost—that suits Glenn to work in the developing world and bonds him with believers like the Walkers.

During a recent trip to California, Glenn visited the Walkers, to see the Project S.A.V.E. operation and give a speech to its supporters.

On a Monday night at a Chico community center, Glenn spoke for more than an hour to a rapt audience of volunteers. He showed scores of photos from missions, and in each one pointed out the medical supplies provide by groups like Project S.A.V.E. "Many of the volunteers were seeing for the first time the patients that benefit from their 'heavy lifting,'" Glenn wrote in his journal. "They said they would never forget the images and stories and were very encouraged that the work they are doing here in Chico is so immediately beneficial in the far reaches of the world. It was a feel-good evening."

The next morning, Glenn joined Janice's regular Tuesday packing brigade at Project S.A.V.E. headquarters, a cluster of storerooms in a self-storage warehouse. "The volume and quality of the stock is amazing!" Glenn wrote. "Large shipments come in weekly, mostly new and surplus equipment, some of it startling in its complexity and expense, all castoffs of American redundancy in health-care technology.

"In the main processing room Janice has flags of some of the countries that have received her containers, thirty-five so far. Several rooms are labeled for the places she sends to most regularly: Papua New Guinea, Belize, Haiti, the Philippines. She has a forklift, she has pallet jacks, she has unlimited boxing and packing supplies. And she has dozens of people on call to come in at any time for packing parties, loading up containers to be shipped off with one final, proud item added, a U.S. flag."

Volunteers who had been in Glenn's audience the previous night brought him supplies they had seen in his photos and knew that he could use. Janice encouraged Glenn to take whatever equipment he could carry home on the plane, even giving him a suitcase to pack it in. Glenn took several items that would prove invaluable on upcoming missions: a suction machine, a blood-pressure monitor, surgical instruments. As excited as a child at Christmas, he chose items to ship onward to far-flung counterparts: sutures and needles, exactly what the Vargheses requested! Oxygen concentrators for his old friend Dr. Edgar Rodas, caring for patients in remote villages of Ecuador.

"It is good to get all these people in contact with each other," Glenn wrote, "and to know that we are all working as one to render assistance."

Janice agrees. At an age when some consider retiring, she's working harder than ever because "the need is so great. When you see it with your own eyes, receive the hugs and smiles from the people who have been blessed by the supplies, the surgeries and the help your group has given—then it takes on a personal face. You long to help, you long to return, you long to give all you possibly can and to help as many as you can. I am sure this desire is what fuels Glenn as well." While the Bible asks all believers to serve those in need, she observes, "Glenn takes that to a level most of us can only dream about."

Pain. As a child, Glenn recognized pain in his mother's limp from her congenital hip dislocation. As an adult, he soldiered through his own pains: divorce, career setbacks, his sons being raised apart. As a doctor, Glenn studied all kinds of pains from every angle—their triggers, their meanings, their management. In time he developed his own philosophy of pain, intricately reasoned and unconventional. He grounded it in the wisdom of a surgeon-missionary he admired, the late Dr. Paul Brand.

With his wife and fellow physician, Dr. Margaret Brand, Paul Brand spent more than fifty years working with people deformed and crippled by leprosy, in India and around the world. He challenged the notion that leprosy itself caused patients' hands and feet to rot or deform. Rather, he concluded, leprosy's attack on the nervous system deprived patients of pain sensations, and without those pain warnings, patients suffered debilitating injuries without even knowing it. While most physicians aspired to alleviate pain in their patients, Brand wished desperately to restore pain in his.

Brand earned international acclaim for the reconstructive surgery techniques he pioneered to address the ravages of leprosy. Later in life, he wrote books (including one titled *Pain: The Gift Nobody Wants*) and continued what he called "my crusade to improve the image of pain." Human beings' ability to feel pain, Brand insisted, "protects us from destroying ourselves." And by accepting pain as an essential element of life, "we can learn to cope, and even to triumph."

Glenn fastened on Brand's philosophy and added his own twists. He would make it a personal goal, he vowed, "to relieve pain in the Third World and restore it in the First World."

In the developed world, "most of us are pretty comfortable," he wrote in an essay. "If we are not, we take all steps necessary to eliminate or relieve the pain. After all, pain is thought to be an unnatural state of events, and we deserve to have a life pain-free." By contrast, Glenn observed, most people in the developing world "don't see a comfortable life as a birthright. They accept life as a painful process, and they have to come to terms with that, without assuming that someone would come along and relieve them of this inevitability."

If the developed world is to genuinely seize its responsibility to the rest of the globe, "those of us who are quite comfortable must be re-sensitized to pain," Glenn concluded. "Sensitization to the human condition requires not just restoration of the ability to experience pain, but restoration of the sense that we must help mitigate it in others." One of the surest ways to achieve that, Glenn concluded, is to take comfortable colleagues on medical missions to the spots where suffering is greatest.

In Glenn's philosophy, it is not enough to observe the world's pain clinically, with detachment or despair that "there is nothing we can do." On Glenn's missions, he calls participants to nothing less than "joyful participation in the miseries of the world."

Of all the social and spiritual phenomena for which Glenn has workable philosophies, marriage has not been one.

Though the decades since his divorce found him mostly married to his work, Glenn still has lamented the lack of a life partner. His three sisters, all long married, worry about whether he is lonely. One of Glenn's standard quips in polygamous cultures is to tell an aging chief with a passel of young wives, "Your example gives me hope!" Threaded through Glenn's year-end letters are references to a few serious romantic relationships, then brief postscripts when each ended.

In 2000, Glenn gave a speech about his mission work at a distinguished arts-and-lectures conclave. There he met another participant, a soprano with a face Glenn found as beautiful as her voice. She approached Glenn to say how much she admired his work. Soon, she was making leading remarks about the two of them joining forces. Though startled by her boldness, Glenn also was charmed and attracted. She seemed eager to know more about his life and missions. He wondered if he might, at last, have found a partner for both.

Within months, Glenn was committed to a relationship with the soprano (then ending the latest of several failed marriages). They rendezvoused when work schedules allowed it; he wrote long letters and e-mails, she much shorter responses. She accompanied him on two missions, organizing music and children's programs while he practiced medicine. Though he had reservations about it, Glenn helped the soprano realize her long-held dream of a land purchase, assisting with arrangements and loans. And he undertook a renovation of his Derwood home to add amenities for a couple: a custom gourmet kitchen, a whirlpool-bath master suite.

Glenn long has been wary of people who aim to give meaning to their lives by borrowing some of his. "I'm not going to graft a soul onto anybody who comes along on these missions" is his standard disclaimer. But he has seen mission experiences have a life-changing impact on participants, and he believed such was the case for the soprano. He believed she shared his mission zeal. He thought she was the love of his life.

Glenn's journals describe month after month of weathering the soprano's emotional highs and lows: distance followed by closeness followed by distance again; messages she signed "I love you" followed by others disclaiming any romantic feelings. Throughout, Glenn was faithful; she, he learned, was not. About six years after their first meeting, she sent a farewell letter informing him she had remarried.

Many who loved Glenn had been telling him for some time, *You deserve better. Forget her. Move on.* Finally, in his journal, he conceded, "They are right." It was a hard admission for a self-described missionary rescuer. The doctor accustomed to saving people now felt, he wrote, that he had "failed to save someone most precious." The healer who took on the pains of the world could not assuage his own.

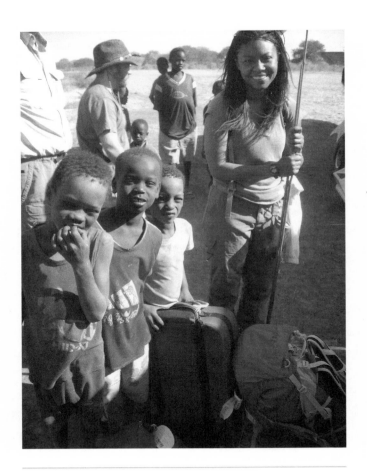

Children in Old Fangak, South Sudan, help carry bags for two members of Glenn's December 2009–January 2010 mission team, public health experts Deaidra Benzing and her husband Adam Benzing (in hat). Deaidra carries a souvenir, a spear made by local tribesmen.

Chapter Sixteen

Transformation

"**Glenn is a collector**," **says his friend Joe Aukward. "It makes** him happy to collect things he finds meaningful": medals and T-shirts from races, artifacts and pen pals from travels, trophies from hunts—and academic degrees. After entering higher education by earning two bachelor's degrees simultaneously, Glenn didn't stop until he had rounded off the diplomas at ten. To his MD degree he added master's degrees in tropical medicine, international affairs, anthropology, epidemiology/public health and philosophy, and an honorary doctorate in humanitarian sciences. Then in 2009 he earned what he swears will be his "terminal degree": A doctorate in education, with a thesis dissertation on the life-changing learning derived from medical missions.

Transformative Learning, a theory pioneered by Columbia University educator Jack Mezirow, describes a particularly potent way that adults learn. The transformative learning process begins with a "disorienting dilemma"— some event that shakes what the student previously had known, assumed or experienced. Through serious reflection and discourse, the student reevaluates old beliefs and frames of references. Ultimately, the process can result in a new, broader understanding of the world and in far-reaching change— transformation—in the student's perspectives and behaviors.

Glenn long has believed that connecting medical students from the developed world to poor patients in the developing world is the ideal setting for transformative learning. He set out to make that case with data in his doctoral thesis.

In the twenty-first century, health care and health-care education must adapt to meet "the increasing demands of a diverse global population across a widening gap in health resources," Glenn wrote. But changing health-care systems requires first changing the global knowledge and perspective of "individual students and practitioners of the healing arts," he contended.

"Ignorance about the health problems of the majority of the world's inhabitants is understandable, since medical education offers almost no exposure to the global population," the thesis continued. "If entry-level health-care students were made aware of the global population in need, they might better appreciate their problems and potentials." When students are guided through the transformative learning experience of an international medical mission, they gain "a better understanding of environments where health-care resources are constrained but health and humanitarian problems abound," Glenn wrote. And, as a result, they become more convinced of both their ability and their responsibility to use their medical skills to serve humanity.

To gather data on how mission experiences affected students, Glenn recruited about 120 premed and medical students who had participated in international medical missions. The students filled out survey questionnaires and were interviewed about their mission experience: Did it increase their knowledge, their confidence, their sympathy for patients, their comfort working in a multicultural environment? Did it change how they behaved professionally or personally, or how they viewed health care and resource allocation? Did the mission's effects soon wear off or, months later, did they still feel changed by what they learned?

The quantitative data showed that on every measure, students believed the experience had strengthened them as medical practitioners. The vast majority also reported that the experience had changed them personally and permanently, prompting them to consider how to build humanitarian service into their future medical careers. Given that the missions were such transformative learning events, Glenn's thesis urged that they be made more widely available to aspiring medical professionals, that they be built into core curriculum and training rotations, and supported with more academic personnel and resources.

Glenn's thesis summarized the study results: "a statistically significant and personally meaningful change in the participants through the international medical mission experience." But the study data only confirmed what he already knew, powerfully and personally, from the stories of mission comrades.

Nearing thirty, Kevin Bergman made a well-considered life change: He left a promising career in business to enter medical school. At GWU, Bergman

Then-medical student Kevin Bergman poses with patients during a medical mission to Malawi in 2003. Now a doctor, Bergman says missions with Glenn were "life-changing," and shaped his decision to found an organization, World Altering Medicine, that raises money and recruits volunteers for needy hospitals in Africa.

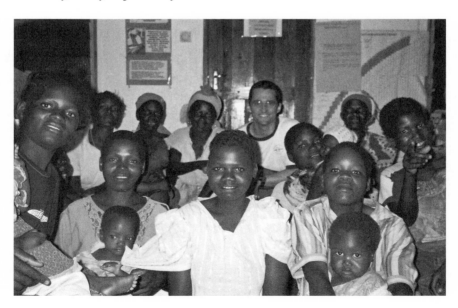

attended one of Glenn's lectures, signed up for one of Glenn's missions, and found his life changed in ways he could not have imagined.

In summer 2001, after his first year of medical school, Bergman joined Glenn's mission team staging clinics in remote villages of Ladakh where doctors rarely ventured. "I felt like I was doing something for the people, but I wasn't really—it was much more for me," Bergman says. "It was opening my eyes to how so many people live in the world, with zero medical care."

During the final clinic of the trip, the long lines of patients included a girl, no more than seven, who complained she could not keep up with the other children. Bergman never will forget the examination. "I stuck the stethoscope on her chest and instead of that *lub-dub, lub-dub* you're supposed to hear, there was a whistling, rushing sound," he says. "I never had heard anything like it. Dr. Glenn listened and said she probably had a hole in her heart wall, what's called a ventricular septal defect."

Surgery to repair the defect was relatively straightforward, Bergman knew, but it was totally out of reach for this child. "Her father was an illiterate farmer with no money," he says. "Going to Delhi to get pediatric cardiac surgery was never going to happen." Bergman huddled with a trip colleague, Sam Gorman, "and we felt like, 'We have to help this person.' Sam stayed on after the mission to help with arrangements. I donated some money and went home, and we raised some more. Mostly because of Sam's legwork and perseverance, we were able to send the girl and her family to Delhi to get the hole in her heart fixed, and she went on to live a normal life. It was really sweet.

"Sometimes you look at the problems of the world and they look so frigging overwhelming. But when we looked into the eyes of that little girl and knew that $2,000 would make it possible for her to live, it seemed so simple."

Through medical school, Bergman kept a photograph of the girl on his refrigerator "to remind me what I was going into medicine for." In 2002, his mission with Glenn was to Malawi; in 2004, it was to Somaliland. "When you have those kinds of experiences in life, the blinders come off and you really see things," Bergman says. "It totally changed me."

Serving his family-medicine residency in Santa Rosa, California, Bergman met a like-minded resident named Dan Dewey. What Bergman had seen while working on Glenn's missions was much like what Dewey had seen while working with pediatric-AIDS patients in Swaziland: people dying in African hospitals for lack of simple, relatively inexpensive medical interventions. In 2006 the two founded a nonprofit organization called World Altering Medicine to raise money for struggling hospitals in Swaziland, Malawi and Uganda, and to recruit medical personnel to volunteer in the hospitals.

World Altering Medicine focuses on cost-effective contributions with life-or-death impact. For example, though oxygen is essential in treating malaria, pneumonia and respiratory diseases that are leading killers of children worldwide, 80 percent of children in Africa who need oxygen do not get it, Bergman says. Since 2009, the organization's Breath of Life initiative has supplied seventeen African hospitals with concentrator devices that need only a power source to generate life-saving oxygen. "We're small," Bergman says of the organization, "but we've got a big heart."

Now a family medicine physician, Bergman chose his current job in a Contra Costa, California, hospital emergency room because it allows him to take off a few times a year to go work in Africa. He says he's acting on what he first learned on missions with Glenn. "The lesson of what one person can do—that's what drives Dr. Glenn so much," says Bergman. "He sees people that 99 percent of the world doesn't see, and he knows that with just a little attention, a little money and surgery and teaching, you can make an enormous change. Once you get infected with that bug, you've got it."

Bethany Larsen recalls the scene distinctly: She was sitting on the couch in her Wisconsin living room at age five, holding her baby brother, Andy.

For more than an hour, she stroked his fine hair and outlined his tiny features with her fingertips as the people from the funeral home waited. "My father ensured that I would be the last person to say goodbye," Larsen later wrote of that day. "I found happiness in the realization that Andy's suffering was over, and, although I was merely five years old, I vowed that I would

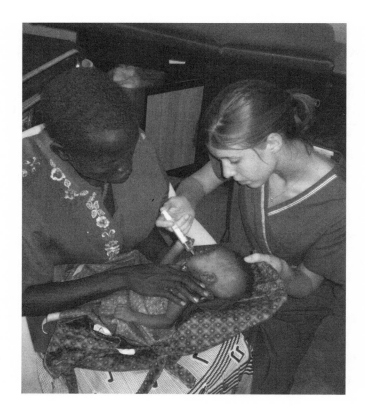

On a December 2007–January 2008 mission to South Sudan, team member Bethany Larsen worked with a distraught mother who had delayed traveling with her infant to the hospital for fear of ambush by tribal enemies. By the time they reached the hospital, the baby had severe pneumonia and could not be saved.

someday cure the leukemia that took my brother from me. Then, I kissed him on the forehead and let him go forever."

As she grew up, Larsen still imagined becoming a doctor, but doubts intruded. The childhood dream of curing cancer probably was beyond her grasp. Why attend long, costly years of school just to wind up working in a stuffy hospital? Was this really the life she wanted? Then the letter arrived, an invitation to the National Youth Leadership Forum on Medicine, a Washington, D.C., program for teens interested in the medical field.

At the final lecture Larsen attended during the ten-day forum, a bearded, live-wire physician described medical missions he led to Africa. Approaching Glenn after the lecture, Larsen learned that the youngest participants in Glenn's previous missions had been twenty-three-year-old medical students. But she and her father, Scott (a veteran of humanitarian work in Bolivia), met with Glenn to discuss possibilities. Four days after Christmas 2007, sixteen-year-old Larsen was on her way to South Sudan with a team that included Glenn, a paramedic, and a half dozen public-health, premed and medical-school students.

Team members were among the first Americans to work in a newly opened health facility, the Duk Lost Boys Clinic. "Lost Boys" was the name aid workers gave to some twenty-five thousand South Sudanese boys who, starting in the mid-1980s, were separated from families or orphaned when government troops destroyed their villages. The youngsters traveled for hundreds of miles over months and years to reach refugee camps in Ethiopia and Kenya. Beginning in 2001, a few thousand Lost Boys, by then young men, were resettled in the United States with church and charity sponsors. One of them, John Bul Dau, told his story in the documentary film and memoir *God Grew Tired of Us*, a story that mentioned Dau's dream of bringing health care to his home village, Duk Payuel.

With friends from the First Presbyterian Church of Skaneateles (New York) that had sponsored him, Dau and other Lost Boys founded the American Care for Sudan Foundation to fund and build a clinic. Glenn had shared a dais with Dau in the United States and was eager to bring a medical team to the Duk Lost Boys Clinic, the only reliable medical facility within seventy-five miles.

During the two-week visit, Glenn's team sponsored a feast to celebrate the new clinic. But for most of the mission, "We labored from sunrise to sunset in the small clinic, seeing hundreds of patients every day," Larsen wrote, in diary entries she would later fashion into a college-application essay. "The clinic was crudely constructed of cement floors, a tin roof, and several plastered rooms on either side of a narrow hallway. Due to the lack of a proper ceiling, bat droppings spattered the walls, cabinets, worktables, and floors in peculiar patterns, and flies and other insects roamed freely."

Supervised by Glenn and other medical personnel, Larsen learned to take patients' histories, give shots and medication, and clean and bandage wounds. During one shift at the clinic, she heard an ear-piercing scream, ran toward it and found a young mother sprawled across the floor in hysterics. The woman's baby, diagnosed with severe pneumonia, lay motionless on the blanket beside her. Larsen picked up the baby and, for an instant, she was again five years old, holding a child she wished desperately to save. Her diary recorded the scene:

Three medical students raced in after me. I held the baby girl as we rapidly checked for signs of life and found a slight pulse. One of the medical students began CPR . . . She did not respond, and there was nothing more we could do. The nurses took the child from my hands to prepare her for burial.

When asked why she waited so long to bring her sick child, the mother replied that she had no choice. It had been too dangerous to travel because the Murle were nearby, attacking neighboring tribes, killing their men and stealing their children. So the mother had waited two weeks, watching her baby become sicker, before making the forty-eight-hour trip to seek treatment.

Before she left, the mother thanked us, calling us "angels" and "blessings from God." I thought of how truly amazing these people were because, despite everything they had been through, they were the most faithful, giving people I had ever met. Despite losing everything to famine, disease, and genocide, they went to church every Sunday, praising God more fervently than the most dedicated Christians in America and giving anything they possibly could to the offering plate. Despite the fact that many times we could do nothing with our limited supplies to cure those who had walked for days to seek treatment, they expressed immense gratitude for the opportunity our presence offered . . .

I left Africa with a drive to succeed far beyond what my imagination previously permitted. One day, I will be a doctor. I will use my knowledge to benefit others. I will be the change I want to see in the world, in Africa. I will live my dream.

As he scouted locations for a January 2008 medical mission to South Sudan, Glenn got word of a new stop his team might make. In the town of Werkok, a shipping container had been converted into a self-contained, temporary operating room. Near the container, in what months before was just an empty field, a 30-by-100-foot hospital was being built, by a charitable group based in Grand Rapids, Michigan! When Glenn e-mailed to learn more, he came away with an inspiring story and an energetic new ally, David Bowman.

A seventy-three-year-old father of five grown children, Bowman calls himself "just an ordinary guy. Graduated from high school, never went to college, learned how to make dental crowns and bridges," then stayed in the dental lab business for fifty years. In summer 2000, diagnosed with heart problems and diabetes, Bowman retired from the lab but immediately was restless. When a Grand Rapids charity advertised for help resettling Lost Boys arriving from Sudan, Bowman and his wife, Nancy, agreed to sponsor five. Three days before Christmas, the Bowmans met their new, seventeen-year-old "sons" at the Kent County Airport.

Two years later, the boys were thriving, but Bowman was not. Doctors found seven blocked arteries and readied him for quintuple bypass surgery. Bowman remembers lying in the hospital bed and thinking, "If I don't make it through this, what will my legacy be, what will stand out in the minds of my kids and grandkids? If I could choose, what I'd want to stand out in their minds was: When God wanted him to do something, he was willing." On the eve of the operation, one of his resettled "sons" had asked Bowman to help bring a Sudanese religious leader, Bishop Nathaniel Garang, to visit Grand Rapids. Bowman survived the surgery and, in his recovery bed, arranged Garang's visit.

The bishop arrived with an assistant; the assistant arrived with a toothache. Through an interpreter, Bowman asked when the assistant had last seen a dentist. *Never,* said the man, who was in his late-thirties. *What about doctors?* Bowman asked Garang. *Surely your people have doctors. No doctors,* Garang told Bowman. *People just come to the church, and I hold their hand and pray for them. Many times I watch them die.*

"It made me sick to hear it," Bowman says. It was, in the terms of Glenn's doctoral dissertation, the classic "disorienting dilemma" that sparks a transformation. Jolted by the reality of suffering in Sudan, Bowman felt powerfully drawn to address it.

In a Bible class where the lesson from Corinthians declared that if one member of Christ's church suffers, "all the members suffer," Bowman blurted out what he was feeling. "As we sit here," he said, "our brothers and sisters in Sudan are dying for lack of medical care. What are we doing about it?

"And then, the thought came to me: 'Bowman, what are *you* doing about it? Are you willing to go?' And I was thinking, 'I have heart disease. I'm a diabetic. I'm not a doctor. I don't know anything about building.' I came home from church and shared this with Nancy and thought she would say, 'You can't go!' But she just sat quietly and made no comment. And I walked away thinking, 'Lord, are you serious?'" Very serious, Bowman concluded, after one of his pastor's next sermons was titled "God Uses the Most Unlikely People."

Throughout 2003, Bowman told anyone who would listen that he felt called to go to South Sudan to explore building a hospital. One by one, Bowman says, "God brought people" both eager and ideally suited to help: Dr. Donn Ketcham, MD, a missionary who had helped build a hospital in Bangladesh; engineer Dave Bixel and his wife, Sandy, a nurse who as a teen lived with her missionary family in Sudan. In 2004, Bowman and eight others visited Werkok, where staggering poverty and virtually nonexistent health care convinced them of their calling. They formed a nonprofit, Partners in Compassionate Care (PCC), and began laying plans for a hospital.

Over the next five years, Bowman and PCC colleagues raised money, recruited volunteers, begged or bought construction materials, and traveled regularly to Sudan. Work was slowed by the months-long rainy season, impassable roads, and unreliable supply shipments. Finally, in April 2009, on Palm Sunday, the Memorial Christian Hospital (MCH) was dedicated. The hospital's director and only full-time MD is a South Sudan native named Ajak Abraham, known to all as "Doctor Ajak."

During the civil war, after troops from the north repeatedly raided his village, Ajak, then nine years old, walked to Ethiopia to join the ranks of rebel "boy soldiers" (though, as Ajak told Bowman, his AK-47 was bigger than he was). Ajak had been a soldier for two years when rebel leader John Garang came to exhort the boys to choose the pen over the gun and become students instead of fighters. Through the Ethiopian president's friendship with Fidel Castro, Ajak was among six hundred boys sent to Cuba for schooling; when he expressed a desire to become a doctor, he got medical training there, too. Then the Christian mission group Samaritan's Purse enrolled Ajak in its Sudanese Physician Reintegration Program, enabling him to complete his MD training in Canada in exchange for his return to serve his homeland. When Glenn's mission team came to MCH in January 2010, Doctor Ajak and his small, minimally trained staff were treating more than 2,100 patients a month.

Though PCC built and sustains MCH mostly with donations from religious groups and individuals, the hospital now raises some funds by charging patients a small sum for care. "I believe MCH is going to be the model for providing health care for all of Southern Sudan," Bowman says. The goal, he says, is that by 2015 the hospital will be self-sustaining and run by Sudanese, especially Lost Boys returned from America. Bowman knows some consider this an impossible goal, "but we also were told it would be impossible to build a hospital in Werkok, and yet there it sits. God did it."

With both Bowman and Dr. Ajak, Glenn felt an admiration and a kinship. The Michigan retiree had overcome his own frailties and doubts to plant healing and hope where there had been little of either. The Sudanese physician had foregone an easier, richer life abroad to come treat and teach his fellow Sudanese. Both followed a path that Glenn also chose and commends to mission participants: opening themselves to the needs of a suffering world and then encouraging and guiding others who would do likewise.

_____

FROM GLENN'S EMBANGWENI, MALAWI, MISSION JOURNAL, JULY 7, 2009:

The one student who gets today's high marks is Jason. He assigned himself to the maternity ward for the first three days here, with the idea that he would not be delivering babies ever again as an internist if that is the residency he completes, so he is now going to do a few. That goal of "a few" was surpassed in his first day, and since then he is awash in the juices that come out of women and the small fry to which they give birth.

On his first day, he participated in more deliveries than his total on the two months of obstetrics rotation at GWU and its affiliates — and the pace has picked up from there. As I write this, he is "between twins," meaning he has delivered the first of a pair in a first-time young mother. He is shaking from hunger since he has not been out of his apron, boots and gloves since arrival on the maternity ward after our morning report. Before the twins, he had delivered four babies, all first-time mothers and several of them big babies.

It is a population explosion such that I told him that in two years if I return, all I need do is call down the children's ward the name "Jason" and a dozen kids will pop up.

Jason Bartsch was entering his fourth year of medical school at GWU when he joined Glenn's mission to Malawi. Bartsch, a Colorado native, previously had worked in emergency medicine, volunteered at a clinic in a low-income area of Washington, D.C., and had gone with medical

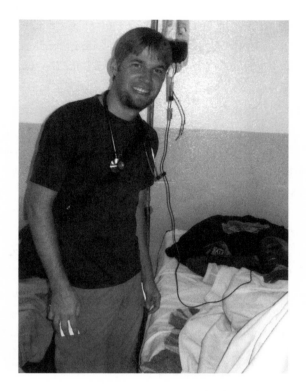

During a medical mission Glenn led to Embangweni, Malawi, when an AIDS patient needed a transfusion, mission participant and medical student Jason Bartsch donated his own blood for the procedure.

teams to Guatemala and Haiti. From those experiences, Bartsch concluded that "it's easy to get caught up in thinking, 'I'm going to provide this care and that care.' But it's important not to forget how much we will learn from them, from appreciating their cultural view and asking for their opinions. It's important to take the 'me' out of it."

That meant, for Bartsch, doing virtually whatever was needed, with guidance from Glenn and Embangweni Hospital staff: first, the exhausting, fruitful days on the maternity ward; then working in the men's ward where, when a late-stage AIDS patient with Bartsch's blood type needed a transfusion, Bartsch sat down long enough to donate a unit, then walked the bag of blood back to the ward.

On the surgery rotation, Bartsch says, "I met a patient that became one of my favorites: an epileptic in his early-twenties who had fallen into a fire and burned his right leg from the knee down and just lived that way for months." Bartsch assisted with the amputation of the part of the man's foot that was beyond salvage. Then, with other mission mates, he spent hours debriding the burn wounds, scraping away dead tissue to encourage new growth healthy enough to take a skin graft. Months after returning from the mission, Bartsch still wondered whether the grafts were a success and the man's leg saved.

In Malawi, as on earlier medical missions, "the people are so great," says Bartsch, now an internal-medicine resident in Vermont. "They don't expect you to come in and cure everything; they're just thankful for any help you can give them." He has heard other trip participants express frustration that they couldn't accomplish more, but he sees it differently. "We might not be curing the world, but we're there helping and working with them," Bartsch says. "I was able to learn new things and to assist the local people and teach some things. And when we left, they weren't left in this big, black hole with no support." The experience strengthened his resolve, Bartsch says, to make missions a regular feature of his medical career.

The best teachers of medical students, Glenn contends, are and always will be patients, especially those "who endure illness, poverty and disadvantage with good grace and courage."

As a teen in Oshkosh, Wisconsin, Gene Wright worked as a hospital orderly so he could watch and learn from his father, an ob-gyn and general surgeon. Wright entered medical school aiming to become a surgeon also until, during his third-year surgical rotation, two things made him reconsider. He didn't relish a lifetime of bending his six-foot-four frame over operating tables scaled for shorter colleagues. And he didn't, in general, like surgeons—at least not what he calls "the stereotypic surgeon personality: They're gunslingers; they're doers; they don't have a lot of patience for subtlety or for being nice to people. When you're a medical student, either that appeals to you or you start to think, 'Well, surgeons really are assholes.'

"In that third year, I discovered two things," Wright says. "That I liked the work of surgery but wasn't sure my body would stand up to it. And that the people I really liked and saw as role models weren't surgeons but pediatricians and psychiatrists." For the past twenty-five years, Wright has practiced child and adolescent psychiatry in Santa Rosa, California, while raising two sons with wife Betsy Hall, a psychotherapist.

As a psychiatrist, says Wright, "I hadn't listened to a chest or done much other than talk to people for more than twenty years when I volunteered for a medical mission to Tanzania in 2006. It was mostly basic, medical-clinic stuff, but I loved going and giving services to people. I loved spending a few thousand dollars on my end to buy medical supplies and finding I could do so much good with them there." On a repeat Tanzania mission, Wright took every opportunity to assist the mission team's veteran surgeon and was reminded how much he loved the specialty.

"I came home from that mission determined to find some way to learn surgery and do medical service, but nobody over here had ever heard of a middle-aged shrink who wanted to cut people open," jokes Wright. "I couldn't just quit my 'day job' with two kids in college, and nobody knew of any training programs that were not full, five-year surgical residencies. Then one day Betsy was talking to a neighbor who said he had heard of 'this guy who loves to take people on rugged missions and teach them surgery.' I thought, 'This might be my chance!'"

Wright e-mailed Glenn to introduce himself; Glenn wrote right back, inviting Wright to join a January 2009 mission to the Philippines, where they'd see many patients needing thyroidectomies and other operations. Wright tried to prepare by practicing sutures on pigs' feet bought at a nearby deli and by reading *Surgery and Healing in the Developing World*, an online textbook Glenn and colleagues wrote. As the trip approached, Wright says, "I was very, very nervous . . . I was going halfway around the world to work with someone I had never met, to do something I didn't know how to do."

Wright remembers day one in the operating theater of the Far North Luzon General Hospital, in the poor and remote province of Apayo, when

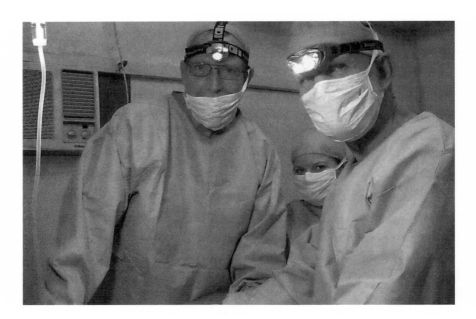

When the electrical power went out in the Far North Luzon General Hospital as Glenn, Gene Wright and colleagues were in the operating theater, the team members moved ahead by the light of headlamps (and an assistant captured the scene in a flash photograph).

he stood across the operating table from Glenn for the first time. "We have prepped and draped the patient for a thyroidectomy. Glenn knows I haven't done surgery since I was a third-year medical student, except for a couple of procedures in Tanzania. I am to assist as he tells me what he wants me to do. He hands me the scalpel, points to the place on the neck to make the incision and says, 'So, try to do it smoothly and all in one motion.'

"It was such a tremendous act of faith on his part. He never had seen me do anything in a body before, and I'm cutting across a woman's neck. I tried not to let my hands shake. I held the scalpel the way they tell you in the book." The initial incision, as well as the rest of the goiter removal, went off without a hitch.

Afterwards, Wright says, "I asked him, 'Weren't you worried about how I might do?' And he said, 'No, because nobody ever cuts deep enough their first time.' And I thought, That's the wisdom that comes from having taught surgical technique to so many."

Thinking as a psychiatrist about his Apayo debut as a surgeon, "Here's how I would read the situation," Wright says. "Glenn talks about people he has taken on missions and encouraged to go beyond what they've done before, and some of them will say, 'This is too much, I don't feel comfortable doing this.' And he understands that is an entirely defensible point of view. But what he knew about me was I was doing this because I wanted to do something new, something outside my comfort zone.

"This is how people learn, under the direction of someone who's done it so many times before. It was unusual only because I was fifty-six and had done psychiatry for thirty years, and we were doing it in the Philippines. Otherwise, he's just the professor of surgery, and I'm just the student of the week."

Like every member of Glenn's teams, Wright was asked to complete a questionnaire about his mission experiences. Wright e-mailed a response that made Glenn laugh out loud:

Dear Dr. Geelhoed,

When we parted company in Manila, you gave me one of your research questionnaires. I filled out much of it there, but left the "essay questions" unanswered until I had returned home to give my experiences time to percolate . . . So now I feel ready to tackle the big question: "How did this experience change you?" with some perspective. And because I know that you sometimes share your students' insights with others (including some who might be prospective recruits), I feel compelled to put my conclusions in the form of some warnings. Ignore them at your peril.

If you are completely satisfied with your professional life, do not under any circumstances meet this man. Do not attend any grand rounds during which Dr. Geelhoed will show beautiful (and heart-wrenching) slides of places you likely cannot find on a map. Ignore the erudite and compelling descriptions of surgeries performed in dimly lit buildings. Pay no attention to the adoring faces that seem to greet Dr. Geelhoed wherever he goes. Be skeptical when he details his yearly travels . . . and don't believe those people who will speak up at these presentations, saying they are colleagues or students who have actually gone with him and SURVIVED these adventures! Predictably, they will even say they "can't wait to go back."

If you are content with all the routines of your life, then you should not plan to meet Glenn at any airport or guesthouse halfway around the world. Don't ride in any primitive vehicles with him, or you may find yourself at a roadside fruit stand, gorging on the tastiest pineapple on the planet. If you're not careful, he may run you along dirt roads (or even stream beds) in search of a village that is always "just a little bit farther," snapping photos the whole way without breaking stride. Never attend a local ceremony with him, or you will soon be enticed to dance with the villagers while your teammates take hilarious pictures that will later be used against you.

I did not heed my own advice. So recently I found myself in a dimly lit OR in the Philippines, standing across the table from this fellow. He handed me the scalpel, seemingly unconcerned that I had not held one since medical school. His confidence was infectious, as was his humor and tirelessness. I cannot believe all that I learned on my aching feet in those two weeks (and all he reminded me that I had not really forgotten).

And the biggest of these anamneses was about being a healer— that a small organization, or a team, or even one person stepping outside his comfort zone can make a difference. I saw staggering need, and felt the rewards of meeting some of that need one person at a time. "GWG" is a teacher, a healer, a raconteur, and a provocateur (and he takes WAY too many pictures). For me he was a catalyst.

Now that I have returned to my "real" life, I cannot stop thinking about when, how and where I will go on another adventure with the good doctor. Didn't I say this was a danger? Don't say you haven't been warned.

Gene Wright, MD
Santa Rosa, CA

Glenn insatiably collects the transformation stories and never tires of telling them. "For me," he once wrote, "this is the international medicine business. My job is I'm the usher; I get people in there. I'm the translator. And then I bring the real experts forward—the locals, the patients—and I get out of the way."

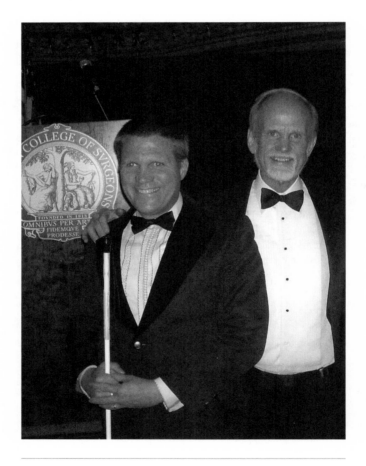

Glenn's longtime friend and running buddy Joe Aukward joined Glenn at the black-tie gala where Glenn received the American College of Surgeons' Operation Giving Back award for his international medical work.

Chapter Seventeen

Giving Back

RELATIVES, OLD FRIENDS, NEW FRIENDS, AND PROFESSIONAL acquaintances; current and former students, current and former colleagues, past and future mission participants. The people to whom Glenn e-mails his journal entries typically fall into one or more of these categories. The cast of recipients shifts over time and by topic; the number of recipients runs from a few dozen to a few hundred. Most who receive Glenn's e-mails say they never can read as much as he writes but try to scan for highlights in the vivid, serialized reports, often sent in batches.

From fall 2009 well into 2010, the e-mails detailed a run of events that epitomize Glenn's life.

FACS. Of all the letters he appends after "Glenn Geelhoed, MD," these are among Glenn's most prized. They mark him as a Fellow of the American College of Surgeons (ACS), the 75,000-member professional society that is the world's largest organization of surgeons.

When the registered letter from ACS arrived, Glenn shared the news in an e-mail headed "THIS JUST IN!" ACS and its volunteerism initiative,

Operation Giving Back, had awarded Glenn a 2009 Surgical Volunteerism Award for international outreach. The award recognizes "those surgeons committed to giving something of themselves back to society by making significant contributions to surgical care through organized volunteer activities," the letter said. Along with six other 2009 award recipients, Glenn would be a featured speaker at ACS's conference in October in Chicago, and he would be honored at an Operation Giving Back reception and a black-tie gala dinner.

Shortly before Glenn left for Chicago, an e-mail arrived from Dr. Andrew Casabianca, a fellow member of the Medical Mission Hall of Fame Foundation board. His nephew's girlfriend, Julie-Ann, a graduate student and aspiring physician, "wants to go on a medical mission to Africa," Casabianca wrote. "I would want her to see it through your eyes and your passion." Perfect timing, Glenn replied: He was setting the final team roster and booking airline tickets for a mission to South Sudan, leaving the day after Christmas. Julie-Ann Cavallo, self-described "Italian from the Bronx," had been on an airplane twice in her twenty-four years when she signed on for the mission. With just weeks to raise trip funds, she dipped into savings and sold white plastic bracelets inscribed with the name of Glenn's web site, MISSION TO HEAL.

The day of Glenn's ACS presentation, running buddy Joe Aukward flew in from Washington, D.C.; sisters Martheen, Shirley and Milly and their husbands all drove in from western Michigan. Before Glenn's speech, they sat outside the conference hall, sharing reminiscences: how, as a child, Glenn hated to swallow pills but learned by practicing with M&Ms; and how, after playing the card game Authors, he decided to read every book in the deck—fifty-two literary classics by the likes of Dickens, Twain and Shakespeare. Glenn's sisters marveled at his memory: "He never forgets a birthday." They praised his ability to persevere despite adversity, a trait modeled by their mother. And in Glenn's gregariousness and love of meeting people, they saw shades of their "glad-hander" father.

Glenn's relatives found seats in the conference hall as Glenn joined the panel of Surgical Volunteerism Award recipients: two surgeons who work in San Francisco, two who work in Afghanistan, one who works in Kenya, and Glenn's old friend Dr. Edgar Rodas of Ecuador. Dr. Kathleen Casey, director of Operation Giving Back, asked the honorees to speak about their motivation, their work, and the lessons gleaned from their experiences. Most spoke for about twenty-five minutes. Glenn spoke, rapidly and earnestly, for nearly twice that long. Clicking through a seventy-five-slide PowerPoint packed with two hundred photos, he showed his fellow surgeons the patients he had treated, the operations he had performed, the diseases he had encountered, and most of all, the impact they could have as medical mission volunteers.

"Perhaps I can introduce you to these people who are my patients," Glenn said, flashing through photos of faces. "Maybe you should learn something about them, because what they already know about you gives them hope. They know you speak a universal language: You speak surgery, something that is immediately and directly understood by them. You bring the healing arts, which are nearly ideally transportable skills across all human barriers: geographic, linguistic, racial, cultural, religious, political . . .

"On the missions I lead, at every operation or procedure there is most typically a First-Worlder like you or me, and then at least two indigenous trainees. You or I never would be operating alone. You and I will be putting tools in the hands of locals, indigenizing skills, doing as much as we can to work ourselves out of this job . . .

"You will learn a lot, maybe more than you ever have learned at any point in your life. But we're not going there for you. We are going to elevate these people's capacities to care for themselves after we are gone . . . This much we can do, so let's begin."

Casey, moderating the panel, thanked Glenn, calling him a "poetic" surgeon as well as a prolific one. After the presentation, several audience members approached Glenn to ask how they might join a future mission, and colleagues who had known Glenn in earlier chapters—as far back as Harvard and NIH— came up to shake his hand. "What a warm and wonderful experience," Glenn wrote later in his journal. He professed to be startled "that I, a young fellow who should be coming to these meetings to learn a few more things, appear to be now considered a senior surgeon with more wisdom to pass on than to be picked up at such a conclave! I am resisting this near-emeritus status."

Though Joe Aukward was reluctant to take time away from work and family, he was touched that Glenn invited him to Chicago. Moving through the ACS events alongside his friend, Aukward perceived Glenn to be "in his ultimate comfort zone, greeting friends, talking about his international mission work." Glenn had loaned Aukward a tuxedo for the gala and jokingly took a "prom picture" of the two of them before heading out to a pre-dinner reception hosted by George Washington University.

Knowing something of the past strains between Glenn and his employer, Aukward was particularly moved by how the GWU crowd received Glenn. "The cheers were genuine, and loud," he says. Surgery-department chair Joe Giordano told those assembled how proud he was to see the ACS honor Glenn's work, and led a rousing ovation. Giordano, visibly moved, also issued an invitation that touched Glenn deeply: He asked Glenn to give a special grand rounds—an annual event called the Paul E. Shorb Lecture—to GWU medical residents the following spring.

At the ACS gala, Dr. Michael Zinner, chair of the group's board of governors, presented Glenn's award "in recognition of his devotion to providing surgical care and education throughout the world. Each year, Dr. Geelhoed assembles up to eight surgical missions, with teams of medical students, residents, and physicians. Over his career, he has led more than two hundred such missions to Africa, Asia, the South Pacific, and South America, and has inspired countless others to take up the mantle . . . His influence on generations of surgeons is vast, both in the United States and across the globe."

Glenn posed for photos with friends including Rodas, and the two laid plans for Glenn to partner on a surgical mission in Ecuador. Along with the accolades, Glenn received an award plaque and a check, which he had asked to be made out to the Medical Mission Hall of Fame Foundation.

"So, life goes on," Glenn wrote in his last journal entry from the festivities. "And with a little help from our friends, we can recognize that there is a point at which we are learning along and suddenly look up and realize that everyone around us has assumed we have been teaching."

Glenn's journal entry for Oct. 24, 2009, details his running in the thirty-fourth annual Marine Corps Marathon. "My time is not a record for any race, and about two hours off the times I scored only ten MCMs ago," he wrote. "But I ran every step of the way, even if slowly, and managed to enjoy it as well."

The next day's entry includes an urgent e-mail, sent by a missionary in the Central African Republic (CAR) near its river border with Congo, and quickly circulated among Diane Downing, Glenn and others who had worked in Assa. Virtually the entire village, "over three thousand people, have been living in the bush for weeks" to hide from the brutal Uganda-based rebels called the Lord's Revolutionary Army, the missionary wrote. "They have had to evacuate their homes, leaving most of their goods behind, only to have them stolen by the LRA rebels, and then having to camp out in the heavy tropical rains and the chilly nights."

Too exposed in the bush and too fearful to go home, villagers of Assa had become refugees, the missionary reported. "We have just heard that over five hundred children, pregnant women, blind people, and elderly began the hike [more than sixty-two miles] through the forest to get to the river... There will be many challenges—everything from how to get that many people across the river in dugout canoes to digging latrines in the area where they will be staying to finding enough food to feed them until international organizations begin arriving with relief supplies... Please pray for all of us involved."

From later, scattered reports, Glenn and Diane learned that a makeshift CAR refugee camp had become Assa in exile, with some five thousand villagers living in tents. Old age had long since silenced Bule, the master drum carver. His son Jean Marco was among the exiles, looking very old and tired. Of countless others, nothing was known.

"So I had six weeks to raise $5,000, which with prayer and busting my tushy I did," Julie-Ann Cavallo says. Cavallo's parents (father Paul is a butcher

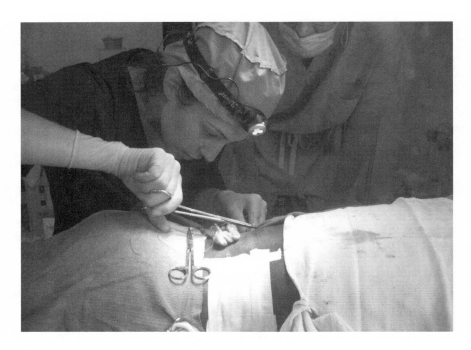

Aspiring physician Julie Cavallo stitches up a patient after surgery during a January 2010 medical mission Glenn led to South Sudan. Cavallo raised funds for her trip expenses by selling plastic bracelets bearing the name of Glenn's web site, MISSION TO HEAL.

and mother Jo-Ann is a computer technician) were concerned that she was putting herself in danger by going on Glenn's mission to Sudan. "But they understand," Cavallo says, "that I'm up for a good challenge." The letter Jo-Ann Cavallo gave her daughter to read when she got to Sudan was full of warnings—"Do not wander alone." "Don't talk politics or religion." "Wash your hands and then wash them again!"—but also encouragement. "You are strong to your convictions and thick-headed to your beliefs," it read. "You will be doing wonderful things for the people of Sudan!"

In addition to Cavallo, Glenn's team included a veteran nurse, a husband-wife team of public-health experts, a documentary-film crew, and psychiatrist Gene Wright, whose college-student son Geoff came along for what was Gene's second mission with Glenn. The documentary crew came to film the story of Dr. Ajak and other onetime Lost Boys now working to improve health care in their homeland. Gene Wright's aim was to help as many surgical patients as possible while assisting and learning from Glenn. Cavallo also was eager to get clinical experience and specifically wanted to treat lepers as she'd read about in the Bible.

Glenn considered the trip critical to advancing an ambitious, long-term vision of his: a network of indigenous medical personnel at South Sudan clinics and hospitals who, after learning new skills from visitors like Glenn, could cross-train each other in those skills.

Glenn imagined this "medical- and surgical-education exchange" network linking facilities where he previously had worked: in Duk Payuel, the Lost Boys Clinic founded by John Dau; in Old Fangak, the operation run by Dr. Jill Seaman, whose work fighting infectious disease was rewarded with a 2009 MacArthur Fellows "genius grant"; in Werkok, where Dr. Ajak runs the Memorial Christian Hospital built by Dave Bowman's Partners in Compassionate Care group; maybe even in Pibor, the Murle tribal stronghold. Because these "networked" hospitals would serve Dinka, Nuer, Murle and other peoples riven by violent tribal clashes and cattle raiding, Glenn saw them as a source not just of care but of leverage: If tribes wanted the treatment and supplies to keep flowing, they would have to pledge to stop fighting.

New Year's Eve found Glenn's team in Old Fangak around a fire ring on the banks of the Nile, watching a lunar eclipse to the soundtrack of ululating voices and AK-47 automatic fire greeting the new decade. A few weeks earlier, Glenn had received an e-mail from Jill Seaman about a burgeoning epidemic of visceral leishmaniasis, a deadly, parasite-borne infection often called by its Hindi name, *kala azar* (black fever). "Glenn, we are in the midst of a *kala azar* outbreak," Seaman wrote. "We are completely overwhelmed. Thus I cannot make a surgical clinic happen . . . I do not know what this will mean for your team."

Glenn's return e-mail assured her, "We will do what needs doing." During the team's six days in Old Fangak, that meant a few emergency operations, helping as they could to manage hundreds of *kala azar* cases, and witnessing firsthand what Cavallo called the "extraordinary and inspirational" work of Seaman, "who has given her life to the Sudanese people."

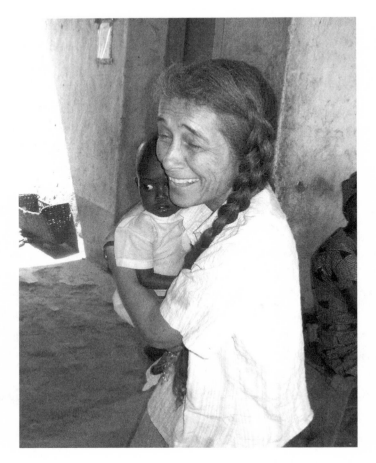

Glenn has led several mission teams to Old Fangak, South Sudan, to the medical outpost run by Dr. Jill Seaman, whose work fighting infectious disease earned her a 2009 MacArthur Fellows "genius grant."

Next stop: Werkok, where Glenn's team and Dr. Ajak's would be learning from each other while handling as many medical and surgical cases as they could in nine days. However, Glenn told his journal, "If I were Ajak, I would hardly be able to carry on activities of daily living let alone hosting the mission which we launch today." The team had walked into a situation as personally taxing for Dr. Ajak as it was fascinating for anthropologist Glenn: the cattle-culture negotiations to win Ajak his bride of choice, Tabitha.

That Ajak and Tabitha loved and wished to marry each other seemed almost beside the point. By Dinka tradition, male relatives would award a bride to a suitor only after assessing all contenders' qualifications, including how many cattle each could produce as a bride price. The cattle would be required not from the groom alone, but also from his relatives and friends, on a sliding scale determined by their kinship and affluence.

Because Tabitha had many suitors and Ajak was a prominent figure in Werkok, the price already was high by the time Glenn's team arrived. "103 prime cows," Glenn wrote in his journal—by Ajak's reckoning, at roughly US$850 per cow, more than US$87,500—plus a sum of cash still being negotiated. "Ajak himself can only come up to almost US$10,000 dollars in the kinds of ransom demanded, and all of his uncles and clan mates must pledge the rest," Glenn wrote. Once the cattle and cash dowry were settled, Tabitha's and Ajak's clans would gather for the wedding celebration. Glenn had promised to buy the bull to be slaughtered for the wedding feast, and the event was scheduled for one of the last days before Glenn's team was to depart.

As the negotiations dragged on, Glenn's team experienced a far more lethal aspect of tribal culture. Hearing gunfire during a morning run with Cavallo, Glenn told her it might just be hunters. But he knew that was not likely, and the truth soon emerged. Murle raiders had come in search of Dinka cattle; Dinka herders had fought back, and an unknown number of Murle had been killed. Seeking vengeance, Murle came again. They killed two Dinkas, whose bodies were brought to the doors of MCH. The casualty reports kept coming: three more Dinka men shot along the road, only one of whom survived. Two Dinka women were kidnapped and interrogated at spear-point. When they could not or would not tell the raiders where the cattle were, they were stabbed repeatedly and left for dead. The one who survived was brought to MCH, where Ajak, Glenn and mission team members assessed her injuries, including numerous chest wounds.

With no chest X-ray machine available, Glenn taught the team the physical signs that confirmed his diagnosis: tension pneumothorax, a build-up of air that had escaped from the lacerated lung into the space around it. Left unrelieved, the condition would obstruct breathing and circulation and cause cardiac arrest. In a developed-world setting, Glenn would have inserted a chest tube. But MCH had neither the tube nor the ability to manage a patient fitted with one.

As a work-around, Glenn showed Ajak where to insert a large-bore needle to release the built-up air. When Ajak did, "the needle hissed and sputtered with the escaping air and immediately the patient improved," Glenn noted in his journal. But the work-around proved insufficient. Late in the day, the tension pneumothorax recurred, and the woman went into cardiac arrest. For an hour Glenn's team tried to resuscitate her, without success.

On what was expected to be the conclusive day for the wedding negotiations, Glenn, his medical team and the documentary crew went to the compound in nearby Bor, where Ajak's and Tabitha's families were gathering. The bride and her parents would not appear until the deal was virtually sealed, but the outcome seemed inevitable. Men in Ajak's clan had begun singling out the dowry cows to be delivered to their new owners. Glenn's bull had been slaughtered, and the women set about cooking the beef, filleting Nile perch and preparing rice and greens. The newly built marital hut had been swept clean and lined with colorful cloth hangings.

Clan elders gave speeches, welcoming the relatives and visitors. Glenn spoke also, expressing his admiration for Ajak, introducing the team members and joking that he would take bride-price bids for Cavallo (who wrote later in her blog, "Boy, would my dad love to have those cows!"). As dusk approached, Glenn's team headed back to MCH. In his journal that night, Glenn noted with satisfaction, "We have enhanced the prestige value of Ajak in our support for him."

The next day, the mission team's final operating day at MCH, Ajak called Glenn: Tabitha's parents had joined the negotiations. The wedding surely was near. Could Glenn come to Bor? Glenn asked Ajak whether the presence of foreigners with cameras might complicate things, but Ajak was insistent.

Glenn returned to Bor with the film crew, eager to witness "the grand finale."
His journal recorded what happened next:

> We arrived to see the congregation of people under the tree at
> Tabitha's family camp had swollen. I welcomed the addition of the
> father of the bride (FOB) and told him I could take some pleasure
> in being a part father to Dr. Ajak . . . and I am glad that the union
> of two such wonderful people can bring us all together. This was
> greeted with applause . . .
>
> At the film crew's request, I pulled them over to interview the
> father then summoned the FOB, who had been in vociferous con-
> versations with his clan members. When he spoke to me, the trans-
> lation was as follows: "If you are a friend of Ajak's, where is my
> dowry from you?? You say you are a friend to both our clans, but
> I do NOT know you, and if I do not know you, then you are here
> as a friend of Ajak's and you must provide us cattle . . . "
>
> I told him that I had already bought the only cow he was going
> to see from me, and I had not even eaten a bite of it while he was
> feasting already on the generosity of the humanitarian friend to the
> many clans and tribes in South Sudan. I said the tribes should do
> less competing to take advantage of each other—particularly the
> gentle and most productive people in service to them, such as the
> medical personnel and the would-be son-in-law to whom he was
> being an excessive burden.
>
> I went to Ajak and saw he was disconsolate. Alone, in a dark
> suit and tie, he sat in the hut to be out of view for a period with
> his head in his hands . . . I put my arm around him and said that

our presence here, far from sealing the deal, had torpedoed it. I said I would support him in any way but not aggrandize this naked gouging and greed, which should be called as it is.

We took our leave (I did have operations to be done waiting back at MCH, after all), making respectful calls at each camp and then tiptoeing out of the increasingly heated grandiose negotiations. They were holding up the culmination of the ceremony we were supposed to be documenting until they could skin all of us as effectively as they had skinned my bull now roasting on the coals.

Arriving back at MCH as evening fell, Glenn led Gene Wright and other mission and local personnel through two teaching cases. The first required only local anesthesia and, as Wright remembers it, went fairly swiftly. The second was a hernia operation on a patient who would need "a spinal": anesthesia delivered to the fluid in the spinal column via a needle inserted in the small of the back.

"Doing the spinal is kind of a big deal," says Wright. "Glenn likes to talk people through it but boy, do they get nervous, and it can take a long time. Time is running out, so Glenn steps in and does the spinal quickly and effortlessly, in no more time than it's taking me to describe it now. The patient is ready. I make the incision and the first couple of cuts. Glenn gets in there, showing how to do a particularly complicated part. Then he leaves the case for the rest of us to finish up.

"I asked Glenn later about the spinal, and he said, 'You know, Gene, what you saw is why I don't do that procedure at the beginning of a mission, because it would discourage everyone. In order to teach, I have to let people struggle through the procedure so they learn. If I did it first, it would make their learning more difficult.'"

The next day, while Glenn's team members said their goodbyes in Werkok, Glenn, Ajak and MCH administrator Jacob Gai headed to the Murle tribal stronghold of Pibor, for a meeting arranged and led by Dave Bowman of

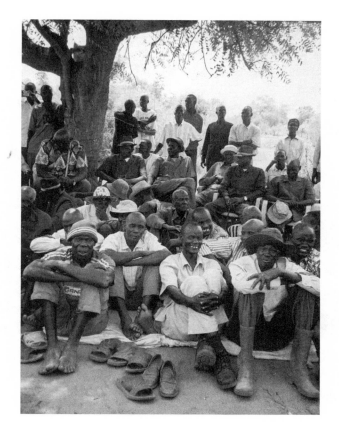

Under the cattle-culture traditions of tribes in South Sudan, Dr. Ajak Abraham could only marry the woman he loved, Tabitha, after striking a deal in which he and his close friends and family provided cash and cattle to Tabitha's extended family. On the day Ajak believed the wedding negotiations to be nearly concluded, relatives from both clans gathered in Ajak's hometown of Bor.

PCC. Bowman would like to see a hospital like Werkok's established in Pibor, where an old hospital building awaits renovation. In the kind of hand-of-God scenario that Bowman loves, the hospital was built years ago in part by missionary Dr. Lambert Ekster, whose daughter Sandy Bixel now is treasurer of PCC. "If we can develop a hospital in Pibor," Bowman says, "maybe God can use us to bring peace and reconciliation."

To the two dozen tribal chiefs at the Pibor meeting, Bowman says, "it

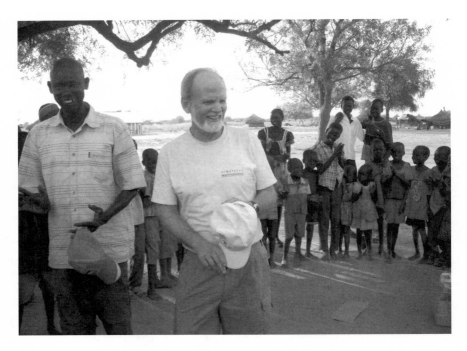

On most missions, Glenn distributes donated clothes, including commemorative T-shirts from races run by his friend and fellow marathoner Imme Dyson. In Werkok, South Sudan, Peter Kuchkon helps Glenn hand out the items.

spoke volumes" that Ajak and Jacob Gai were there—Dinkas coming into Murle territory to discuss promoting health for all. To the government officials attending, Glenn and Bowman made their intentions clear: They would help recruit aid groups to renovate the hospital, and they would help lead medical missions and train medical personnel to work in the hospital—but only if the tribes, in return, would stop attacking each other and seek peace. When Bowman returned to Pibor two weeks later for a second meeting, some participants still sported the tokens of goodwill Glenn had left: Cavallo's white plastic bracelets inscribed MISSION TO HEAL.

(Months later, Ajak would e-mail the outcome of wedding negotiations: "The number of cows is 218, plus Sudanese pounds equivalent to US$10,000. My wedding did not take place yet, but it will soon, I have to finish the remaining amount of cash needed by my in-laws first." In the meantime, Ajak wrote,

"I am really very excited for the next educational event of the 'South Sudan Mission Network,' we are waiting for that great moment . . . Professor Glenn, your team has been a blessing to MCH always.")

On the plane leaving Africa, Glenn wrote in his journal, "I will have a circumnavigation to think about these further details and ramifications of what we have continued in some sites, begun in others, and made plans for in still others." As the rest of the mission team returned to the United States, he flew the opposite direction, to Asia.

After a dozen trips to the Philippines with missions organized by the non-profit group Medical Ministry International (MMI), Glenn's January 2010 visit felt like a homecoming. On the drives to remote hospitals on the islands of Leyte and Mindanao, he stopped at his favorite roadside stands to buy pineapple. As always, the islands' high rates of hypothyroidism meant that goiter patients were lined up at the hospitals, awaiting his arrival. He posed for photographs with two "and promised I would come back to do the same posing after each had been relieved of the goiters."

Also on the mission was Dr. Tricia Moo-Young, an endocrine surgery fellow from Chicago who had approached Glenn after his American College of Surgeons speech and asked how she could work with him. To prepare for the trip, Moo-Young read Glenn's journals from previous Philippines missions. So she knew to expect power outages, came armed with a headlamp, and, when the OR went dark, cheerfully joined in the singing of "This Little Light of Mine."

At the hospital in Tboli, Mindanao, Glenn spent time with a family of fellow volunteers: Janice Walker, whose Project S.A.V.E. provided the spinal-anesthetic kits he just had used with Ajak in Sudan; her husband, David, an ENT surgeon; and the Walkers' granddaughters, Lea Lippert, 15, and Lindsay Lippert, 18. "I envy this three-generation visiting family," Glenn told his journal.

Janice Walker says her granddaughters "loved to hear Glenn's many stories. He was warm and welcoming to them as to all the mission participants, and a nonstop educator in the operating room" where the teens were allowed to scrub in to observe. Both were affected deeply by their time in Mindanao, Walker says—not by just the exciting hours in the operating room, but also the quieter time spent with poor, sick and orphaned children. The mission experiences played a big part in Lindsey Lippert's choice about college: Starting in fall 2010, she would study nursing.

"How is it that I happen to know the distinguished former minister of health of the nation of Ecuador? When first we had met, we were probably not so distinguished and were more like the peripatetic students who accompany me now—searching abroad for a goal that will no doubt turn out to be found within themselves . . . " As Glenn prepared for a February 2010 mission to Ecuador, he retraced history in his journal.

In early 2010, Glenn joined his old friend Dr. Edgar Rodas, the former health minister of Ecuador, for a mobile medical mission to remote parts of that nation.

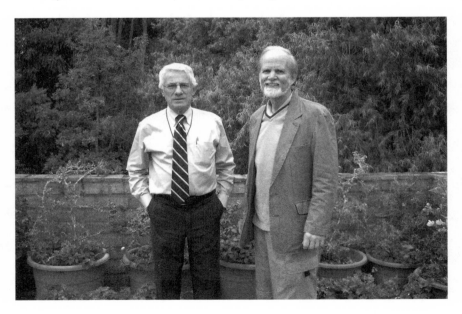

Thirty years earlier, crossing the Pacific Ocean, Glenn stopped on the island of Saipan to see a surgeon-turned-photographer friend, Jack Hardy. "Jack had wanted me to meet a kindred spirit and his wife, who would go out to lunch with us at a pleasant spot overlooking the Pacific as we talked of future dreams. The young man wanted to be a surgeon to the poor people of the world since he came from a country which had so many of them. He introduced himself in good English: 'Hi, I am Edgar Rodas from Ecuador.' "

The two stayed in touch as Rodas rose through his hometown University of Cuenca to become professor of surgery, then dean of the medical school. In 1990 Rodas founded the nonprofit Cinterandes Foundation to promote human development by meeting basic needs, starting with health care. Cinterandes' inaugural project was a mobile surgery program: a truck containing a fully outfitted operating room that visits the most remote corners of Ecuador, where Rodas' team provides surgical care at no charge.

Rodas is justifiably proud of the program's track record. "We've been in seventeen of the country's twenty-four provinces. We've done more than six thousand operations with no mortalities so far and an acceptably low rate of complications. We deliver surgery of excellent quality and in a human way, close to the people in the places where they live." Rodas personally has gone on all of the mobile surgical missions except for two: one when he was ill, and one when his mother died. And that includes the period from 1998 to 2000 when he was working fulltime as his homeland's minister of health.

During the Surgical Volunteerism Award events at the ACS conference, Glenn and Rodas finally set a date: Glenn would join Rodas' mobile surgical team for the last week of February 2010. Glenn planned to bring along one more volunteer, University of Toledo medical student John Lazarus, who had gone on two of Glenn's Sudan missions. Then came the February 7 e-mail from Alex Nguyen, a Drexel University fourth-year medical student who had followed Glenn's work. "Are you going anywhere in the future?" Nguyen asked.

On Feb. 12, Glenn e-mailed back: "How about as soon as February 21-28 on a mobile surgical mission to Ecuador?" Nguyen's swift response: "Yes! Holy mother of God, I would love to go Ecuador with you . . . I called my folks to send me my passport. How much did it cost you to get the ticket and everything? How much cash should I bring? And how do you do surgery in a developing country?"

Nguyen spent his childhood in a Vietnam prison compound where his social worker mother helped rehabilitate women jailed for prostitution after the Vietnam War. "Growing up in that setting, I was exposed to many things that seemed wrong and unjust, and that began my interest in doing something to help people," Nguyen says. He moved to the United States at age twelve, excelled at math and went to college planning to be a bioengineer. But after reading *Mountains Beyond Mountains*, the story of global health pioneer Dr. Paul Farmer, Nguyen realized medical service "is what I want to do with my life." The air force paid for his medical school so he owes them several years' service, which he hopes will be in remote settings where he can use what he learns from Glenn.

On Glenn's medical mission in Ecuador, a post-operative patient is transferred from the Cinterandes mobile surgical unit by medical student volunteers, operating room technician Freddy Peralta (second from right) and Cinterandes driver and assistant Gonzalo Matute (right).

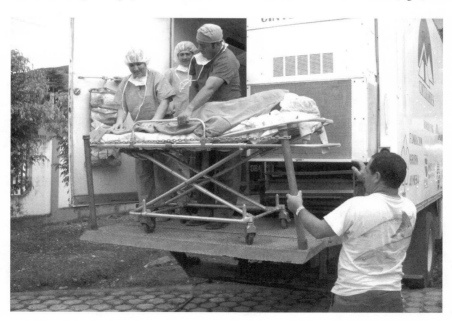

After long hours of international flights, Glenn, Lazarus and Nguyen joined Rodas and other volunteers for the winding drive from Cuenca to the mobile surgical mission destination: Zumba, a quaint town in the Andean highlands near the border with Peru. The Cinterandes truck was parked by a municipal building temporarily converted to staging and recovery space. Rodas, Glenn and colleagues carefully screened patients, choosing only the surgical cases they felt could be done well in the mobile OR and managed safely in recovery once the team departed.

For two days, team members operated until after dark. Patients were borne on stretchers from the municipal building, raised by a hydraulic lift into the OR truck, and swiftly routed through operations including hernia repairs and gallbladder removals. For Glenn, it was a welcome break from the worst of what he'd faced in Africa. "We are dealing here with the rising Second World, not the entropic collapse of the Third World," he wrote in his journal. "This is not surgery on the cheap and making do with what little can be offered. The mixed group of students, from Ecuador and England as well as the United States, is taking full advantage of the opportunities that come from both an American and South American professor of surgery in a tight, full-time tutorial. It is a great experience for all!"

Rodas concurred: "It is beautiful to have somebody like Glenn with us. Of course, we make an exchange of experiences in the surgical field, techniques of operations, but also an exchange of different human experiences." On the mission's final night in Zumba, town leaders threw a banquet and toasted the surgical team with a local home brew of fermented sugarcane juice.

Before leaving for the states, Glenn stayed briefly in a guesthouse at the Rodas family compound, on a lovingly landscaped acre beside the Cuenca River. Rodas and his American-born wife, Dolores, live in one house; a son and his family live in another; and a daughter and her family in a third. On the lawn, the grandchildren have fashioned a miniature golf course. To one side, in a quiet copse of trees, Rodas built a small altar, where flowers surround three burial urns containing the ashes of his father, his mother, and a sister. Someday, Rodas told Glenn, his ashes will be here too. "I told him I hope that it is a long way yet in coming, but I envied him his plans," Glenn wrote in his journal.

A few weeks home from the mission, Nguyen sent a reflective note to Glenn:

> I keep thinking about Ecuador. You know, a doctor isn't complete until he finds his patients. I think I have found mine. I felt like a new world of possibilities has been opened for me . . .
>
> You mention gifts from the poor in the surgical e-book you edited. I think humility is one of those gifts. Despite my background, I felt entitled and ignorant in front of these patients. I felt foolish at the time, not knowing about things like leishmania or leprosy, things that could be part of someone's daily life but I will never see in the Unites States. I had this fear of going into somebody's country with good intentions and end up making things worse due to my ignorance . . . But thanks to you, I learned that sometimes you need to "just do it."
>
> Best,
> Alex

Late in March 2010, Glenn hosted his largest "packing party" ever. If all went according to plan, all the medications, equipment and supplies he could get to Toledo would be loaded into a cargo container there for delivery, months later, to Werkok. Then Dr. Ajak and Glenn could distribute the supplies to the "South Sudan Network" hospitals as part of future missions and training events, starting as early as February 2011.

To help with the packing, Cavallo and other mission alumni descended on Derwood. They sorted, inventoried and boxed up supplies stacked high in Glenn's two basement "mission control rooms." They loaded 140 large cartons into a Penske rental truck, then several team members caravanned with Glenn to the University of Toledo. Once there, they made presentations about their mission experiences during a weekend of events surrounding the Medical Mission Hall of Fame awards presentation.

The awards are given annually to individuals or organizations "that have made significant and substantial contributions to advancing the medical well-being of their brothers and sisters throughout the world," says MMHOF president Larry Conway. Past inductees include Dr. Albert Schweitzer (posthumously), Dr. Paul Farmer, Dr. Jill Seaman and Dr. Glenn Geelhoed. Among those inducted in 2010 was a veteran community health nurse and educator who spent twenty years serving in the Congo: Diane Downing.

⁂

April 2010: Glenn gives a globe-spanning "grand rounds" lecture to GWU medical students and entertains relatives at Derwood while organizing his next missions. May: He hunts turkey in Maryland, runs a 25K race in Grand Rapids, and collects a humanitarian award at an International College of Surgeons meeting in Denver. June and July: On a lengthy trip to Tanzania, he runs the Kilimanjaro Marathon, takes a safari through the Serengeti, and joins University of Toledo and GWU students on missions in rural provinces, where they train locals in surgical technique.

In August, he travels to Burma to provide medical care for internally displaced people victimized by the Myanmar military junta. In September, he returns to Ecuador for another mission with Dr. Edgar Rodas. In October, he hosts friends at Derwood when the American College of Surgeons' annual conference comes to Washington, D.C. In November, he returns to Malawi and then, as ever, Glenn spends Thanksgiving with the Schaefers.

While the last few Christmases found Glenn preparing for imminent departure to Africa, the next trip there would be delayed a month to accommodate what he considers a crowning honor: an invitation to lecture at The January Series, the celebrated speakers series of his alma mater, Calvin College.

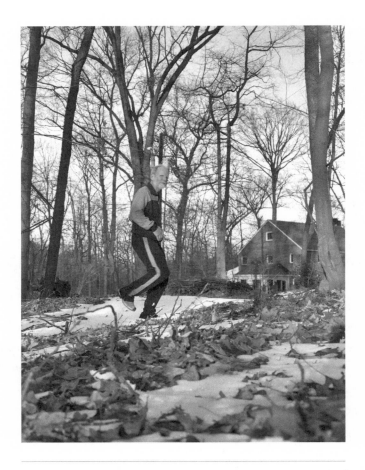

Glenn's home and haven between travels is a property he calls sim-ply Derwood—9.3 wooded acres in the Washington, D.C., suburb of Derwood, Maryland. Glenn savors the property in all seasons.

CHAPTER EIGHTEEN

Derwood

NO MATTER WHERE MISSIONS TAKE GLENN, THE RETURN IS ALWAYS THE same: to the wooded Maryland property he calls simply Derwood.

As Central Park is to New York City, Rock Creek Park is to metropolitan Washington, D.C.: an urban preserve, 1,800 wooded acres laced with streams and running trails. At the headwaters of Rock Creek, in the quiet Maryland suburb of Derwood (population 17,251), realtors in 1976 showed Mary and Dave VanderHart and Glenn Geelhoed a one-of-a-kind listing: 9.3 acres of pristine land surrounding a quirky, custom-built house.

Glenn was sold on the place before he even entered the house. The trees are oak, cherry, maple, dogwood, tulip poplar and hickory; some old giant oaks are a hundred feet tall and ten feet around. Thickets of native mountain laurel dot the hilly lot, which falls as much as thirty feet from the high point where the house stands to the stream-carved valley floor. The narrow, curving Butterfly Creek runs from one side of the property into the wide, boulder-strewn Mill Creek, and then both become Rock Creek, flowing south through Maryland and the District of Columbia to meet the Potomac River. Everything Glenn saw drew him back to his childhood, hunting, fishing, exploring.

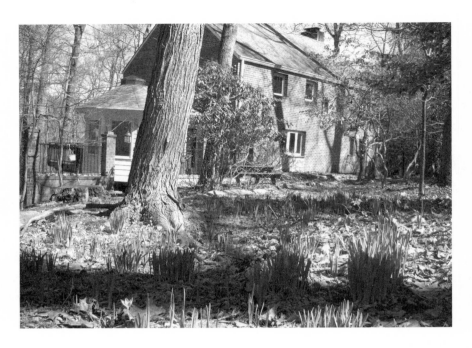

The red brick house in Derwood, Maryland, that has been Glenn's home since the mid-1970s.

But Glenn liked the house, too, not least because it came with a story. Its builder, Lowell Bennett, was a scientist, an expert in applied physics. In the 1950s when Bennett carved a small lot out of the woods for a home where he and wife, Ellen, could raise their family, he designed the house to take whatever nature could dish out. For the exterior walls of the two-story, four-bedroom colonial, he sandwiched three layers: wood framing, cement block and red brick. Bennett knew better than most that no home design could defy the laws of physics. But he could very nearly defeat them, with sixteen-inch-thick walls and two-by-twelve-foot rafters supporting a steeply pitched roof that would withstand strikes from even huge falling trees.

The naturalist in Glenn loved the acreage. The scientist in him loved the sturdy house. The single parent in him longed to provide the kind of rooted childhood that the Bennetts' four children had enjoyed there. In August 1976, two Geelhoeds and three VanderHarts moved in. Michael Geelhoed and Laura VanderHart would grow up as siblings, with Dave and Mary caring for Michael during Glenn's absences. After Michael finished college and moved out, so did the VanderHarts; Michael remains close to the family and grieved with them in June 2010 when Mary lost her life to cancer.

Glenn is eager to show off Derwood. He hosts out-of-town friends and relatives, entertains medical colleagues, treats guests to narrated walks by the creek. But for most of the time he's in town, Glenn is alone at Derwood—in a sense, alone *with* Derwood, a place that serves as not just as the setting of his life but essentially as a character in it. Derwood is Glenn's haven—in *Gone with the Wind* terms, his Tara: a home base between travels and a restorative, Edenic refuge. It is also both headquarters and archive for his medical missions, signs of which are everywhere.

Because he may be traveling for 30 to 40 percent of any given year, Glenn has made an art of buttoning up the house when he departs, putting it in suspended animation. Before leaving recently for a weeks-long mission, he has turned off extra lights and nonessential appliances. About all that's left running are the refrigerators and freezers, and the state-of-the-art security system. It is so fine-tuned, Glenn has been told, that an alarm could be triggered by the transit of a spider.

On this day in the dim and quiet house, a large black spider is blessedly distant from the security sensors. It is clinging to the cement wall of a basement storage room, which, for months, was stacked almost impassably with boxes. This is the "mission control room" where Glenn stores the medical supplies donated by his supporters and "scroungers." When the supplies overflowed this room, Glenn began stacking them in an adjacent bedroom and nearly filled it also.

Since the Penske truck caravan bore the accumulated supplies away for shipping to South Sudan, both rooms are almost empty. In the bedroom, cartons no longer crowd the weight bench where, each morning that he is home, Glenn performs ten bench presses of a barbell equaling his body weight. In the "mission control room," all that's left are a few new donations that have come in and several blue duffels tagged in Glenn's tidy handwriting. "Laji Varghese, Surgical Mission, Himalayan India," says one. Another is marked simply, "Ecuador."

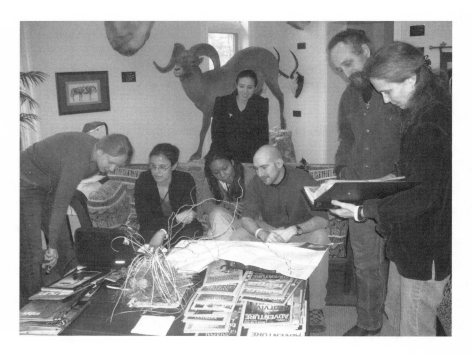

A "packing party" at Glenn's home before the December 2009–January 2010 mission to South Sudan involved friends and relatives as well as participants bound for the mission, including Julie Cavallo (standing behind couch), Deaidra and Adam Benzing (seated in front of Cavallo) and Kathy Shiring (far right).

An anthropologist surveying the rest of Glenn's basement might guess several different hobbyists and professionals live here, all of them wildly prolific. Fishing rods and tackle are bunched in the rafters; guns and tribal blades are secured in safes. In a dusty photographer's dark room, more than one hundred slide carousels line the counter. Shelves full of children's balls and sand pails back up to a wall of files—forty-one deep drawers containing academic papers and presentations. Across from those files, a long bench is scattered with boxes of hunting ammunition, a block of deer food and a well-pierced dart board. The basement refrigerator is stocked with Gatorade and other sports drinks. The basement freezer is full of labeled parcels— ELK BURGER, DEER TENDERLOIN, ELK SIRLOIN—and fowl with feathered wings still attached.

On an aging world map, thickly clustered pushpins mark destinations a globe-trotter has visited—but only through the late 1980s, after which, Glenn says, he didn't have enough space and pin colors to plot every trip.

At the bottom of the basement stairs, mounted on a wall plaque, is a set of dark-tipped, flaring horns from a Nigerian Fulani bull, a souvenir of Glenn's first medical mission to Africa. At the top of the basement stairs is a pantry stocked with canned soups and vegetables, jars of applesauce, boxes of Tuna Helper—Middle-American staples chosen chiefly for their long shelf lives.

Around the corner is the room where Glenn is likeliest to ridicule himself to visitors. *A man of simple tastes, a man who's often gone, a man whose greatest spending sprees are funding medical missions—does he really need a custom kitchen? Granite counters, cherry cabinets, top-of-the-line Viking appliances?*

At first, Glenn was too stung to joke about the costly Derwood renovation that feathered a love nest the soprano never inhabited. But time has passed. Now he points with curatorial pride to the artistry in the hand-painted Italian-tile mural above the six-burner stove. And the Viking fridge stars in a yarn Glenn loves to spin: At 2:30 a.m. on Labor Day 2005, he got a call summoning him to join an emergency-medical team deploying to New Orleans in the aftermath of Hurricane Katrina. He sleepily opened the quarter-ton appliance and, because it had not been properly reinstalled since a service call, it fell over, half-pinning him in a space under the unit and its mangled door. He emerged from under the Viking "wearing a couple dozen smashed eggs" and made it to the C-130 transport plane for the Katrina relief mission. Later, while Glenn changed his scrubs in the New Orleans hospital, the other medical volunteers with whom he was billeted gasped when they saw his full-torso bruises and heard how he acquired them.

To one side of Derwood's kitchen is a hexagonal, sky-lighted breakfast room, with four light oak chairs around a matching table. The table is perpetually set with warm-hued stoneware plates, floral-patterned glasses, and cloth napkins in sunflower napkins rings. Glenn rarely disturbs it between guests' visits and, after serving a meal there, resets it the same way.

Through one door from the kitchen is Glenn's living-dining room. Chairs

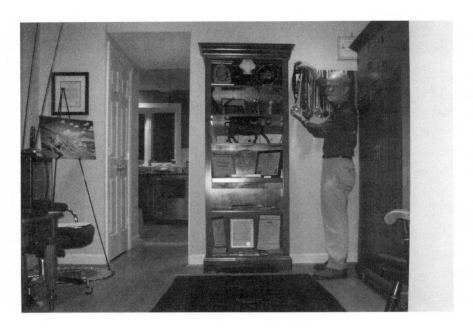

In a small room next to Glenn's home office, awards and certificates he has received fill a tall cabinet, and dozens of race medals hang on a long rod.

and couches surround a low ottoman laden with coffee-table books—about Ecuador, Africa, Sudan, Kilimanjaro—and in-flight magazines from Ethiopian Airlines, Philippines Airlines, Qatar Airways. Through another door from the kitchen are two small, linked rooms that serve Glenn as den, office, library and award gallery. From a long rod on one wall hang dozens of brightly ribboned medals from marathons and other races. A cabinet displays race certificates and academic and humanitarian awards including the stylized bust of Washington that came with the *George* magazine honor, and the sculpted crystal from the Medical Mission Hall of Fame induction.

In Glenn's office, floor-to-ceiling, dark-wood bookcases surround a dark-wood desk. On the wall behind his desk hangs the mounted head of a trophy Dall ram he shot in the Brooks Range of Alaska. On the desktop, among the books and papers, are several stacked towers of coins—a very low-tech security system, Glenn admits with a chuckle, but something he's left for years to reveal any tampering with his desk in his absence.

The library, like half the rooms in the house, holds a portion of the vast Geelhoed archives. On every trip he has taken since medical school, Glenn has kept notes and journals. The records are written in a tiny hand or typed in a two-fingered, hunt-and-peck style (the latter especially since 1993, when he got his first IBM ThinkPad notebook computer). The collected written works now run to thousands of reams of pages and hundreds of CDs (plus countless floppy disks and other now-obsolete formats). For decades, Glenn has been incorporating journal entries into text-and-photo scrapbooks. His methodology is established: Captions are handwritten on pages next to photos of scenery, wildlife, colleagues, operations, patients, and the gory specimens that the operations have removed from the patients. The pages are organized in two-inch-thick vinyl binders, which Glenn buys ten at a time. On this day, he has run out of binders until more arrive in the mail; the pages to fill them are already prepared and stacked on the library floor. Shelves nearby hold several dozen of the newer-vintage binders, with dates and destinations noted on their spines: 2010, South Sudan; 2009, Malawi; 2008, Afghanistan . . .

The rest of the completed binders threaten to overtake an upstairs guest bedroom, where Glenn's sister Milly quilted the bed coverlet with squares of commemorative T-shirts from Glenn's races. Two walls of shelves hold 176 binders, with another fifty-four in rows on the floor. On top of the shelves are three large glass fishbowls and one small glass aquarium, filled to the brim with matchbooks collected on world travels.

Derwood's upper story has two other bedrooms. In the small bedroom: low shelves of medical books with titles such as *Current Surgical Diagnosis and Treatment* and *Pathology of Emerging Infections*; a desk laden with cameras and documents; a ninety-six-drawer cabinet full of photographic slides; a twin-sized bed, spartanly made. Glenn sleeps here. In the large bedroom: a handsome, queen-sized sleigh bed with a rich-looking comforter; a fan on the ceiling and silk prints of Balinese dancers on the walls. Glenn does not sleep in this master suite, which he furnished to please the soprano. For the longest time, he also avoided the master bath's fancy, jetted tub. But after a particularly grueling Marine Corps Marathon, sore muscles trumped bruised feelings and he put the tub to use.

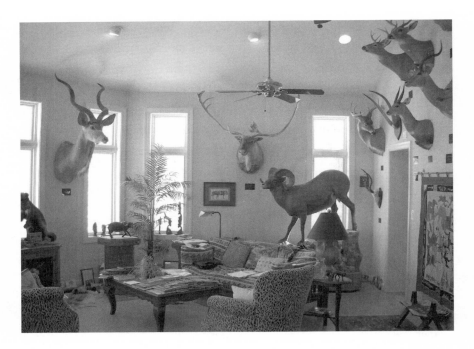

Of all the rooms at Derwood, Glenn's favorite is the cathedral-ceilinged game room, where he displays several dozen hunting trophies: birds and animal heads, skulls and tusks, hide rugs and "full body mounts"—entire taxidermic creatures including a wolverine from Alaska and a Kamchatka snow sheep from Russia.

Of all the rooms at Derwood, the cathedral-ceilinged game room is Glenn's favorite. Through the tall windows and series of skylights, he can see in all directions into the woods, to watch browsing deer, hunting raptors, falling rain and leaves and snow. Inside the airy room, he is surrounded by what he calls "crystallized memories": trophies from his hunts, mementos from his travels, and photos of himself with family.

Animal-hide rugs are spaced so closely on the game room floor that paws touch: red fox, timber wolf, Russian brown bear. So-called "full-body mounts"—entire taxidermic creatures posed on bases mimicking their habitat—include a wolverine from Alaska, a Merriam's tom turkey from Nebraska, and a Kamchatka snow sheep from Russia. Some three dozen other trophies—birds, animal heads, skulls, tusks—are hung on walls or from the ceiling, with bronze plaques giving the genus and species and hunt details of each.

The coffee table is paved with copies of the magazine that first inspired him, *National Geographic*. Window ledges hold collections of wooden figures, carved busts and animals. Around the room's perimeter, propped against baseboards are framed photos of Glenn on missions, Glenn on hunts, Glenn with grandchildren. A strand of cobweb clings to the frame of one of the oldest photos here, of a young, smiling Glenn on a 1960s-style couch, with one arm around Donald and the other around Michael.

At Derwood, even when Glenn is away, he is present—palpable in everything here that speaks to his work and life. Something similar could be said, Glenn hopes, at the sites of his medical missions—that after he has gone, some meaningful trace of him remains: the words of instruction and encouragement to those who would be healers; his hand on a shaking hand, guiding it deftly through a procedure; the shove into "the deep end of the pool" where students gain experience and confidence; the immediate, restorative gift of surgery; the infinite, transformative gift of learning.

"There is a lot of very diverse world out there that needs healing," Glenn once wrote. "Among its inhabitants are many poor, indigenous people who, rather than being overwhelmed by despair at the huge burden of illness and lack of resources, set about doing something about it. These are people who have almost nothing—and are more than willing to give it all in hospitality to those who come from affluent areas of the world to help. These 'gifts from the poor' have taught me and my students much about the spiritual richness of people who may seem to be so impoverished. They do not just survive, but thrive. They sing; they dance; they celebrate life.

"Contact with such patients is not only an inspiration for the idealistic young," he concluded, "but is a sure cure for the jaded veteran who may have forgotten why he or she got into the healing arts in the first place."

Laid out in a corner of the game room, to be addressed upon Glenn's return, is paperwork for his next round of missions. On a ledge nearby sits the tiny, prized possession: Bule's hand-carved drum, as resonant with meaning as when the gift was given.

Acknowledgments

"Give me just a few minutes," Glenn Geelhoed said to the poorly clad man who had approached him in the cafeteria of the George Washington University Medical Center. The man took a seat and waited patiently through my lunch and conversation with Glenn—which, of course, took more than "a few minutes," as do most conversations Glenn has with most people he meets. There are so many stories to tell, each one leading to another; there are countless cross-references, footnotes to footnotes. Our supposed "exploratory meeting" about collaborating on a book became a crash-course introduction to a remarkable life.

Psychiatrist Gene Wright, one of many alumni from Glenn's medical missions, has observed that Glenn "sometimes thinks he's just blending in, but he is always the largest person in the room." In that lunch crowd full of lab coats, there was no shortage of medical credentials. There doubtless were other achievements represented, too: marathons run, mountains summited, books written, awards and diplomas amassed. But only at my lunch table, I suspect, were so many of those feats present in one trim individual—who, as he had promised, rose after our meeting to walk the poorly clad man through the cafeteria line and buy him a sandwich.

My role in this book project has been what Glenn calls "the art of précis": trying to distill the adventures, aims and lessons of his life into a single book. I left our initial meeting imagining that the project would be neither quick nor dull. I was right on both counts. The collected works of Glenn Geelhoed are quite literally countless because just when you've taken a count, he sends more: more journals, more essays, more photos. More hydra-headed e-mails, encouraging his globe's worth of contacts to get to know each other.

I am indebted to many of those contacts. Glenn's sons and sisters were especially insightful and generous with their help. So were several hunting and running buddies, longtime colleagues and veteran mission participants. I thank them for their invaluable contributions to getting the story right. And finally, I thank Glenn for inviting me along on this adventure. It has been a privilege to share, through this collaboration, in the gifts Glenn's patients have given him and the worthy work he gives back.

—PATRICIA EDMONDS

                                   ·

AT SOME UNREMEMBERED MOMENT IN THE PAST, I IMAGINED (FALSELY, as it develops) that attempting to perform operations without adequate resources, consuming foul water and rancid food, running a marathon in inhumane temperatures, or being trapped by a blizzard while studying antlers on a mythic bull elk—I imagined that these were challenges. These are, I now know, sheer delights by comparison to writing a book dealing mostly with one's self.

Were it not for Patricia Edmonds, this book would still be a scatter of notes, photographs, letters and memories littering the Internet, my attic and my mind. Patty began as a well-recognized collaborator and became a trusted friend. Her patience, persistence and professionalism, and her ability to reduce my ramblings to the shape and size of a digestible morsel, are all impressive. Her capacity for listening is boundless. She writes with the purity of an angel's soul. Had she been or done anything less, this book would still be an idea.

Wise and steadfast friends have lent time, knowledge and insight to shape this book, chief among them Diane Downing, Craig Schaefer and Joe

Aukward. Special thanks are owed to esteemed colleagues at George Washington University including Drs. Paul Shorb, Joseph Giordano and John Williams, and Professor Peter Hotez—men of courage and decency, each of whom has made signal contributions with far too little recognition. Some miles to the west, Larry Conway and Dan Saevig at the Medical Mission Hall of Fame Foundation and the University of Toledo have supported this project since its inception. I'm indebted to each of these good people.

The longer we labored over the telling of this story, the more I recognized how important to me had become the many fellow travelers on international medical missions. Some were colleagues who gave endlessly of their skills and their time. Some were young and largely inexperienced; of these, many imagined themselves to be my students. Ultimately, all became my co-learners and, in some memorable instances, my instructors. What each of us would confess is that the real teachers were the patients and those who loved them. They honored us with permission to enter their lives and trusted us before we had given them reason for trust.

Dust had collected on some of the memories revived by Patty's incessant questioning. She coaxed me into bringing back stories I'd nearly forgotten and people I now realize did more to shape my thinking, and my life, than I had earlier realized. I was irritated when she pressed me to visit events I'd chosen to seal in the vault of forgetfulness, grateful when she led me back to childhood and family, to early lessons that became life values, and to sisters whose affection can never be fully acknowledged. And I was impressed, again, that what matters most to me is that I have been given two sons, Donald and Michael, men of character and accomplishment with families of whom no father or grandfather could be prouder.

Thea Joselow and Erik Dunham have for some time lent their superb talents to the design and development of *MissionToHeal.org*, the web site where the story begun in this book continues to be told tribe-by-tribe, mission-by-mission, day-by-day. My thanks to each of them.

And what do I say of those thousands of people, perhaps tens of thousands, the heroes I've met in places of beauty and brutality around the globe? Local healers who knew the power of a root, a leaf, a plant that Western medicine has not yet imagined; trained physicians and committed nurses, families and neighbors, pastors and strangers—each of them demonstrating that the grace of human compassion is the fountain of life and healing. I am in awe of these women and men for whom healing is never a burden, for whom day-and-night service is a passion and an apparent joy. When they speak to me of their hopes, I hear the echo of a more ancient voice whispering about "the least of these, my brethren." In their drive to learn and apply new learning, they bring me back to Tennyson's conversation with a "Flower in the Crannied Wall."

> *Flower in the crannied wall,*
> *I pluck you out of the crannies,*
> *I hold you here, root and all, in my hand,*
> *Little flower—but if I could understand*
> *What you are, root and all, all in all,*
> *I should know what God and man is.*

In the wake of the little I have learned and done, I see throngs of women and men whose labor, love and humility inspire me to repack a worn bag, throw another file of memories into the attic, and go again. If I appear driven, I am, in fact, called—and I hear the call in their many languages.

They are God's flowers, roots and all, who have most nearly opened my mind to "know what God and man is." To them, I dedicate this book—as, earlier, I dedicated my life.

—GLENN W. GEELHOED, MD